Living with Cancer

Living with Cancer

Ernest H. Rosenbaum, M.D.

A Frank E. Taylor Book

PRAEGER PUBLISHERS   New York

Published in the United States of America in 1975
by Praeger Publishers, Inc.
111 Fourth Avenue, New York, N.Y. 10003

Library of Congress Catalog Card Number: 75-4342

Printed in the United States of America

This book is dedicated to my wife, ISADORA,
my companion in life and assistant
in medicine, a woman whose daily efforts
have enhanced the quality of my life and
given comfort to both my patients and me,
and to our patients, who have taught us
so much about the meaning of life

Contents

Acknowledgments

I wish to thank Tina Anderson, who has been my literary editor and worked for a year with me, my patients, and their families to capture an accurate pulse of what it means to be living with cancer. I also wish to thank Henry Bean for literary assistance in the initial phase of this effort.

I received invaluable medical reviews from Myron R. Blume, M.D., Joseph Bottino, M.D., Carol Fellows, M.D., and John V. Siebel, M.D.

For general review and assistance I want to thank Sylvia Douglas, Mary Kahn, Julius R. Krevans, M.D., Margaret M. Mahoney, Faneuil J. Rinn, and Mark Zborowski, Ph.D.

Anna Vikart generously assisted with the typing of the manuscript.

I am also indebted to Dr. Cicely Saunders, O.B.E., F.R.C.P., for allowing me to describe her excellent work at St. Christopher's Hospice.

Living with Cancer

It is impossible to make all of the sick well, for the physician in that case would be superior to the Gods: but the physician can secure respite from pain and intervals in disease and can render disease latent. One must be fertile in expedients and not be satisfied to apply his mind entirely to the writings of others.

—Aretaeus the Cappadocian,
second century A.D.

Introduction

Being told you have cancer is like being hit by a truck. In a few seconds the course of your life is altered. You can only ask the unanswerable, "Why me?" If the cancer is advanced, you are tormented by questions of how long you will live and how much you will suffer. You wonder whether you will be able to endure pain and maintain your dignity. You wonder what the end will be like.

It is hard to imagine feeling more isolated or racked by anxiety than you are at that moment. Yet unless you can share your thoughts with someone who is compassionate and candid, but also knowledgeable about cancer therapy, the anxiety and sense of isolation may increase. You may neither find comfort nor be shown a pragmatic approach to your problems. Instead, you will probably sense embarrassment and fear in those around you, a subtle pressure that prevents you from speaking of your deep concerns.

Undergoing diagnostic tests and therapeutic procedures can reinforce the feeling that you are no longer in control of what happens to you. You are poked, prodded, questioned, and tested, and may feel ashamed of a new dependence on your physician and others. At the same time you may agree to almost anything in your fight to survive.

When such anxiety accompanies disease, the result can be a patient who does not respond well to medical treatment and who withdraws into a deep depression, too bewildered and frightened to function in any area of his life. It is the purpose of *Living with Cancer* to describe how such debilitating emotional reactions can be prevented, or worked out creatively, through a reciprocal relationship based on an exchange of thoughts and information between patient and physician. In defining such a constructive relationship I have drawn on my own successes and failures and have tried to describe the techniques and approaches that have worked for me and my patients.

I want to present here my philosophy of life as well as an approach

3

to medical treatment. Other doctors will have equally valid approaches to the treatment of cancer. This book is primarily for patients and their families, written with the hope that they will see the value of open communication with their physicians and other members of the health team, and that they will be able to participate in a medical treatment that combats their disease and diminishes their suffering. But because of the void that sometimes exists between physician and patient, this book may also be helpful to those in the medical professions. A candid, mutually helpful relationship can be created only between two willing participants who both understand the benefits to be gained.

In beginning to penetrate the immobilizing terror that cancer causes, my first concern is to make sure a patient understands that I want to offer personal as well as medical support. We approach his problems together, whether his disease is curable or potentially fatal. I am interested in everything that concerns him—his work, his family, his sex life—for if I can free him from excessive worry, he may not only respond better to therapy but also have more desire and energy for the things he enjoys.

I ask each patient to enter into an unwritten contract with me. The terms of the contract call for candor between us at all times, for mutual trust, and the understanding and assurance that I will control any pain he may have in the future. Faith in the continuation of this agreement is what ultimately lessens his anxiety and allows him to turn his thoughts to living.

But cancer is not a single disease, and how well a patient lives will be determined by the kind of cancer he has as well as his particular psychological makeup and his body's response to treatment. Each patient is unique, and so is the course his disease will follow. One person will be cured; one with residual disease may obtain a remission or may have a subsequent recurrence; the disease of another may become stable with neither regression nor progression; and still another will eventually die of his malignancy. At present about 33 percent of cancers are cured,* but practically all cancers are treatable. Even if cancer invades certain organs, it may not be serious unless it causes functional impairment. The essential problem is not that one has cancer and that it has spread, but whether the cancer will respond to therapy. The answer to that question may not be evident for weeks or months. Until time has passed after surgery or with other treatment, one cannot be precise in predicting success or failure. Thus with any cancer therapy one needs time and medical reassessment to measure what has been accomplished, what has been gained or lost.

* The American Cancer Society's *1975 Facts and Figures* states, "Of the 665,000 new cases, 220,000 will be saved."

People used to speak of five-year cures and ten-year cures, but this is not an adequate definition. Some cancers are cured at once, usually by surgery or radiotherapy, and some are never cured. Certainly after five to ten years a patient may have a high-percentage chance of having been cured, but the accuracy of such a pronouncement will depend on the type and stage of cancer. What is needed, therefore, is comprehensive testing at regular intervals for all patients for many years. Such a statement is not meant to create anxiety about the possibility of a recurrence. Rather, it is intended as an additional safeguard, even in cases where there is a high probability of cure.

The unpredictability of the course any malignancy will follow and the uniqueness of each patient's physical and emotional responses to treatment are the reasons why most physicians will not attempt to reply to the question "How long will I live?" These are also the reasons why a patient with advanced cancer can have realistic hope of obtaining remission and a good quality of life.

Some of the patients described in the following pages have been cured; others have died. All of them willingly shared for the purposes of this book their private thoughts and feelings in the hope that their experiences, good and bad, would provide a yardstick of how life may be lived under the limitations imposed by cancer.

I hope, therefore, that *Living with Cancer* will convey some of the frustrations, emotional and physical, a cancer patient may encounter, and offer ideas on how to minimize those frustrations. Part I, "The Unwritten Contract," describes the general patterns of diagnosing and treating cancer and some of the anxieties associated with these processes. Parts II through V consist of chapters on the thoughts and experiences of individual patients, with special emphasis on what cancer can do to a person's self-image and on the supportive role of the family. Part VI offers information about the many people and services, in and out of hospital, that are devoted to supporting cancer patients and their families.

Part I
The Unwritten Contract

1 · A Diagnosis of Cancer: Telling the Patient

A young man once came to me after knowing for nine months that he had a testicular mass. He had postponed consulting a doctor because he suspected he had cancer and felt this would prevent him from providing for the financial future of his family. By this delay he had forfeited the possibility of a cure.

A person may put off consulting a physician for many reasons, chief among them the fear that his suspicions will be confirmed. But whatever the reasons for postponement, recriminations from the doctor only increase remorse. When physician and patient meet, it is time to get to know each other and to discuss the procedures to be followed in obtaining a medical evaluation of the illness. It is time to forget past omissions and to concentrate on the present and the future.

Of course, not every person who consults a physician about a perplexing ailment suspects or assumes that he has cancer. But because I am a hematologist and an oncologist, concerned with the study and treatment of blood and tumor problems, most of my patients are referred by other doctors and therefore are usually aware of why they are consulting me. Some are referred by their family physicians when cancer is suspected; others are referred by internists, surgeons, or cancer specialists for re-evaluation and further treatment. But for whatever reason and at whatever stage in his malignancy a person reaches me, a candid exchange of information must be made in our first meetings. A new patient is always apprehensive, so I try to provide him with the basic facts about cancer and its treatment while he relates his symptoms and some of the personal facts about himself that I need to know as his physician. I believe that an informed patient will be more receptive to treatment and thereby improve his chances of combating his disease. Moreover, the attitudes he acquires in these initial interviews may well affect the quality of life he is able to maintain for the duration of his illness.

9

At this time a routine medical history is taken and a physical examination and appropriate diagnostic tests are performed. Arrangements are also made for any necessary surgical, medical, or radiation consultations. A patient is always kept informed about why a particular test is being performed and what the results could mean. False hope and disappointment would only make him distrustful of me and wary of future treatment.

Patients should be aware that they are entitled to all information about testing, test results, and therapeutic procedures. In California the right of an individual to "informed consent" is delineated in the State Supreme Court decision in Cobbs v. Grant, handed down in October 1972.* Patients in California now read and sign in the presence of their doctors an "informed consent" for special diagnostic procedures (such as angiograms), surgery, radiotherapy, and experimental chemotherapy and immunotherapy. Appendix I contains a Patient's Bill of Rights approved by the American Hospital Association in February 1973, and Appendix II shows a copy of an "informed consent" form that I use in my practice. This provides the minimal necessary consent, and of course it protects the physician as well as the patient.

A full evaluation usually takes several days because of the necessity for diagnostic procedures, additional consultations, and possibly surgery. Occasionally, it may even take several weeks to establish a diagnosis. Of course the slightest delay will seem interminable to a person who has been worrying alone for weeks or months.

In very rare circumstances a diagnosis may have to be postponed. One of my patients had had fever and enlarged lymph nodes. Three biopsies had been performed before he was referred for consultation for a possible lymphoma. A fourth biopsy was performed and reported as a lymphoma, but additional tests and exploratory surgery had negative results. A dozen pathologists and cancer specialists reviewed his slides without arriving at a unanimous conclusion. The patient, whose disease has not progressed, has been observed for over a year instead of being treated. So far he has suffered no recurrence, but he is aware that he may have cancer and understands the reasons why we prefer not to institute therapy until a firm diagnosis is established.

Fortunately, misdiagnoses are the exception. In Mort Segal's case (see Chapter 5), a rare malignancy was misdiagnosed as benign until, nine months later, what was thought to be a cyst was excised and proved to be malignant. Misdiagnoses do not often occur these days because questionable slides are routinely sent to pathology consultants

---

* Those who want to find out the legal definition of "informed consent" in their own states should check with the state medical society or an attorney.

around the country, a procedure that represents an additional safeguard for the patient. It was only the extremely rare nature and the difficulty of pathologic interpretation of Mort Segal's malignancy that led to the delay in diagnosis. Most cases are not complex.

How I tell a patient he has cancer depends in part on how many previous conversations we have had and on whether he has just undergone surgery. If I do not know him well, I may begin by asking him what he knows about his condition or what his other doctors have told him about it.

Knowing that what I say may affect the rest of his life, I proceed slowly and carefully, ready to temper my approach as he reveals how much he wants to know at that moment. It is, after all, a patient's prerogative to choose how much he wants to hear. I, however, must be sure I have provided the opportunity for him to find out everything he wants to know. Many patients now bluntly ask the question "Do I have cancer?" But if a patient tells me to take over, that he does not wish to know the details of his disease or his treatments, I do not usually press the issue. He may know his limitations and function better at the level he has chosen. The only people I believe must be informed more fully than they indicate are those responsible for the support of others. Of course, such delicate maneuverings are unnecessary when a patient has made a previous request to be told exactly what is found.

Naturally, when a patient has just undergone surgery I wait until he is strong and lucid enough to deal with any potentially shocking news. I usually sit beside his bed to create a sense of informality. Doctors often seem so busy that a patient feels guilty and apologetic for taking up their time. Since I too have a heavy schedule, with many interruptions, I plan serious discussions for late afternoon or early evening, when there is less chance of interruption as well as adequate time to reply to all of a patient's questions.

When possible, I prefer to have the closest family members present at the time of the explanation. This eliminates the need for repetition and reduces the possibility of misunderstanding. Sometimes, too, the inclusion of the people he loves lessens a patient's fear of abandonment and reassures him that his family is not concealing knowledge from him. Together the family and the patient can ask questions and consider problems that may arise in the future, for, ideally, the long-term treatment of cancer involves the cooperation of the whole family. The benefits to a patient of such a supportive family are apparent in the chapters on Darrell Ansbacher and Magdalena Matunan.

A patient can be much more helpful—and much better informed—

if he will supply answers to a doctor's leading questions to keep the discussion open. When a doctor asks, "Are there any questions about your diagnosis?" he will be stymied by a reply of "No," or "You're the doctor. You should know." As I mentioned in the Introduction, the doctor-patient relationship works best when both participants are mutually responsive. For example:

"What do you think is wrong?"

"I'm not sure."

"Well, there are several possibilities. Acute infection or arthritic or systemic disease—or some other type, an ulcer or a malignancy. What do you think is causing your problem?"

"I really don't know. Can you tell me?" or "Do I have cancer?"

When the reply is, "Yes, you have cancer," or "Yes, you have a tumor," a detailed explanation should be given, repeating much of the basic information the patient may have received during diagnostic procedures. He should be told the type and extent of his malignancy, although not necessarily all at one time; and, most important, he should be made aware of the treatments that are available to combat his disease. I always explain that we will begin with the mode of therapy prescribed for his form and stage of cancer but that there are others which may be equally good or provide a backup if the first one is not effective.

However, a patient is usually too stunned to think clearly and needs time to assimilate the bad news. Often he cannot respond to my final question, "Is there anything you don't understand about your problem?" He may understand nothing because he has heard nothing since the word "cancer," or he may be so confused that I conclude the interview and promise to return later in the day or early the next morning. I always suggest that he make a list, which I call the patient's "shopping list," of all the questions that occur to him about his particular form of cancer, future treatments, or anything else that worries him, no matter how unrelated it may appear to be. This will help him to include thoughts he might otherwise suppress.

Occasionally a family member will intervene and request that a patient not be given his real diagnosis. My feeling is that any agreement concerning a patient should be between the patient and the physician. When a patient comes to me for medical help, it is with him that I make a contract, although I do, as I have indicated, welcome support and prefer that the family be informed and take part in discussions with the patient.

The wife of one of my patients made a request for secrecy. She eventually admitted that she felt guilty toward her husband and might subconsciously have assumed responsibility for his disease. With another patient, I suspected that his wife wanted to play a dominant role in her husband's illness. She offered as an excuse for withholding information her belief that her husband was psychologically incapable of handling the truth. Such a supposedly weak patient is usually stronger than anyone thinks and is quite capable of dealing openly with his cancer. In both cases I convinced the wives that their husbands would cooperate more fully in their therapy if they knew about their disease. At other times, when the psychological impairment of a patient has been a reality, I have given limited information.

The reverse situation has also occurred. I have had patients request that their disease be kept secret to protect a spouse or other family member. In these cases I try to explain to the patient the therapeutic advantages of treating a family as a unit. For instance, a husband who joins his wife during an office visit will share her problems, know about her fears and her therapy, and therefore be able to offer invaluable backup support. I had one patient who would always tell me she felt great until her husband interrupted with "That's not true. You've had . . ."

Of course, everyone has heard of instances when a family member and the patient each thought he was alone in knowing the truth. Again, I feel I can and should play a positive role by bringing them together.

Sometimes the circumstances are even more difficult. I am occasionally brought in on a case in which the deception of a patient has been going on for some time. The family or the primary physician made an early decision not to tell the patient the truth, so the question arises of the wisdom of intervening in an established relationship. My policy in such cases is that if a patient has no psychiatric problem, and if he asks me directly, I tell him about his disease in as much detail as he wishes. But if he shows no inclination to know about his illness, I tend to comply with the wishes of the family and the primary physician, even though such a policy has many times brought unfortunate results.

In one such case I had a patient with advanced cancer, with lung involvement. Her husband, a powerful, domineering man, was adamant about not telling her of her illness. Throughout their marriage he had protected her from every unpleasantness; now he would protect her from the knowledge of her cancer. Against my own judgment and advice, I deferred to his wishes because I was afraid my interference would create a situation that could be emotionally damaging to a structured marriage of over thirty years.

In accordance with instructions from her physician, who had known her for many years, and the concurrence of her husband, I told the woman she had an inflammation and instructed the hospital staff to be discreet in her presence. After exploratory surgery and chemotherapy she was released and went home, but as her disease progressed, she gradually deteriorated and naturally wondered why, although her husband repeatedly assured her everything would be all right.

One evening she was admitted to the hospital for further therapy. Her husband was sitting with her when the medical resident visited her room to obtain a routine history and physical examination. She was frightened and in pain. In an effort to reassure her the doctor said, "Don't worry. You're in the hands of one of the best cancer doctors in San Francisco." The woman screamed and burst into tears. Her husband collapsed in his chair with chest pains. Fortunately, an emergency electrocardiogram and medical evaluation did not reveal the suspected heart attack, but the woman lost confidence in me and subsequently would believe only a part of anything I or her husband told her. She became depressed and angry, even more distrustful of her husband than she was of me. She died several weeks later.

We betrayed this patient, first by concealing the truth and then by failing to provide adequate protection from the truth, although I always felt she suspected she had cancer, as most patients do. If she had guessed her real condition before she died, she could not then have avoided feeling the same resentment and hurt she had felt upon hearing it from a stranger. But, more significantly, perhaps she might have planned her final months differently if she had known she was going to die.

The ambivalence of my feelings in this situation is obvious; but I do not feel that I, as a consulting physician, have a right to reverse such a critical decision unless the patient brings the matter up with me.

Of course, a patient who does not know he has cancer presents other, practical problems to a physician. The diagnostic and therapeutic procedures involved in most types of cancer are usually so complex that a patient is bound to worry about why such procedures are necessary for a simple infection. One does not easily explain away the need for radiation or drugs that may cause severe reactions. I have found it easier to take care of a patient who knows he has cancer, who understands its implications and is willing to endure the side effects of therapy in the hope of obtaining improved health.

2 · Cancer Therapy

Surgery, radiation therapy (X-ray or cobalt), and drugs (chemotherapy) are currently the three mainstays in the treatment of cancer. Using one or a combination of these treatments, physicians are able to effect a definitive cure in about a third of all instances where a malignancy is diagnosed. Obviously the cure rate for some types of cancer is much higher, and for others much lower, than this average. It is important to note here that, while treatment fails to cure approximately 67 percent of the patients, it is rare that vigorous treatment does not materially benefit the patient. Even in cases when it is obvious from the outset that cure is unlikely or impossible, adequate therapy can assure the patient not only freedom from pain, but many additional months to years of relatively normal life. It is surprising how often one encounters a nihilistic attitude toward the treatment of cancer, not only among patients and the lay public, but even within the medical community. This is often summed up as "If it cannot be cured, why bother treating it?" It seems strange that such thinking persists in a society in which the treatment of other incurable diseases—heart disease and diabetes, just to name two—is readily accepted.

Because the currently available treatment often fails to effect a cure, physicians and other scientists are continually developing new and experimental therapeutic approaches to cancer. Unique combinations of the three anticancer therapies mentioned above, known as multimodality therapy, and experimental immunotherapy are examples of recent innovations. Experimental approaches to cancer treatment obviously undergo lengthy testing in the laboratory and upon animals before being introduced into human medicine. However, eventually an experimental

* This chapter is meant to provide only the most simplified description of cancer therapy. No attempt is made to indicate a preferred method or to give details of a specific modality. Those who want further information should ask their physicians.

treatment reaches the stage where it must be "tried out" in cancer patients. Such patients are always given a detailed explanation of the reasons why their doctor feels that an experimental treatment is justified in their case. It is worth emphasizing here the unwritten law that an unproved experimental therapy is never used on any patient for whom there exists a tried and effective alternative treatment.

Many people have heard frightening stories about the side effects of treatment, both conventional and experimental. These stories make them more afraid of therapy than they are of cancer, but such fears are largely unwarranted in the multimodality approach to cancer. Through today's sophisticated diagnostic and therapeutic techniques, major pain and suffering can be reduced, alleviated, or prevented altogether.

Surgery

Surgery offers the ideal primary approach to the cancer problem. If you can "cut it out" without major functional impairment, and there is no residual disease, you may effect a cure. Surgical excision is appropriate when a tumor is localized and does not involve vital structures. Normal function can be maintained after the removal of a kidney or part of a lung. In some cases a biopsy is performed at the start of surgery and the tissue is examined by a pathologist who immediately reports his findings to the surgeon. If there are no malignant cells in the tissue, the surgeon can perform a conservative or limited operation to remove the suspicious mass. If the tumor contains malignant cells, the surgeon can immediately perform an operation designed to eliminate all traces of the malignancy.

Frequently a surgeon is able to remove all visible evidence of the cancer, thus presumptively effecting a cure. However, depending on the type and stage of the tumor, in a certain percentage of cases cancer will recur, either adjacent to its original location or at some distant site, such as the liver, lungs, brain, or another organ. This hallmark of cancer, its tendency to spread before the parent tumor is diagnosed and removed, constitutes the single greatest problem in the management of malignant diseases. Thus after the operation one must have close medical follow-up and wait several months or years before there is a reasonable certainty of cure.

Early diagnosis is the prerequisite for a successful cancer cure. Unfortunately, except for cancer such as that of the cervix, for which we have a Pap smear, physicians lack routine techniques for diagnosing cancer at its earliest inception, when the likelihood of its having spread is minimal. New tests are becoming available, but until they are perfected, most cancers will grow for months or years before causing symptoms that will lead to their detection by physical examination, X ray, or biopsy. In the meantime, the obvious symptoms a person can identify by himself are often ignored, despite the public education program of the American Cancer Society* and the public statements of many cancer specialists. Whether this postponement is due to fear of cancer, of surgery, or of therapy, delay may only allow cancer to spread, often precluding cure.

Radiation Therapy

Certain tumors, such as cancer of the cervix and Hodgkin's disease, may be cured by radiation therapy. Hope for many cancer patients not cured by surgery may also lie in this mode of treatment. It is not a last resort, as many people think, but a practical method of killing cancer cells, restricting growth, or reducing a tumor to a size at which surgery becomes a practical possibility. The most likely candidate for radiation is the patient with localized cancer. When cancer has spread, radiation may also be used to alleviate pain and other distressing symptoms.

In radiation therapy, protons, electrons, or other charged particles are aimed directly at a tumor. The effect of the radiation beam is to damage the genes, the DNA, of the tumor cell. Such damage usually makes the tumor cells incapable of further growth and division. It is impossible to avoid some damage to normal cells in the path of the radiation beams, although normal cells are generally more resistant to damage than tumor cells. To minimize this problem as well as to obtain the most efficient results, the normal tissues are shielded as much as possible and the recommended radiation dose is spread over a period of time. The area of treatment, depth of dose, and tissue tolerance, as well as side effects, are considered when the mathematical calculations are made for the individual patient. New techniques are being developed that will further reduce the damage to normal cells. In the meantime, improved equipment and safety techniques have, for many patients, lessened or eliminated some of the side effects of treatment, such as skin burns, nausea, vomiting, and diarrhea.

---

* The seven danger signals, as listed in the American Cancer Society's brochure "Listen to Your Body" are
   C   Change in bowel or bladder habits.
   A   A sore that does not heal.
   U   Unusual bleeding or discharge.
   T   Thickening or lump in breast or elsewhere.
   I   Indigestion or difficulty in swallowing.
   O   Obvious change in wart or mole.
   N   Nagging cough or hoarseness.

Chemotherapy

Chemotherapy is the treatment of a malignant disease with drugs that attack and may destroy cancer cells. It is generally reserved for systemic cancers and cases in which surgery and radiotherapy are no longer effective. An exception is the use of chemotherapy as an adjuvant to surgical treatment. Here drugs are administered for their prophylactic effect. For example, experimental adjuvant chemotherapy may be administered immediately after surgery for breast cancer (when cancer cells have been found in the adjoining lymph nodes). This is done in the hope of eliminating undetectable or microscopic foci of cancer cells in the body and thus postponing or preventing a recurrence of the disease. In a few diseases, such as Burkitt's lymphoma, choriocarcinoma, ovarian cancer, leukemia, and some cases of advanced Hodgkin's disease, some cures may be achieved by the judicious and aggressive use of chemotherapy alone or in combination with other modalities.

Like healthy cells, cancer cells are involved in a continuous process of resting and dividing. It is characteristic of cancer cells that, unlike healthy cells, they divide in an uncontrollable manner and invade normal tissues. Chemotherapy takes advantage of our knowledge of the cyclic life pattern of cells. The chemotherapeutic agents are cellular poisons, which are classified as noncell-cycle specific, cell-cycle specific, or miscellaneous, depending on their mode of action.

The noncell-cycle specific class of drugs, the alkylating or mustard group, may attack all the cells in a tumor, whether they are resting or dividing. These drugs reduce the tumor mass. Then the remaining cells may be activated toward cell division. Since many cells are killed more easily during the process of division than when they are resting, the cell-cycle specific class of drugs, the antimetabolites, are used to attack the cancer cells during the phase of cellular division, when they are more vulnerable.

As with radiotherapy, it is virtually impossible to attack cancer cells with drugs without affecting normal tissues as well. The normal cells in the body are also dividing, and those that divide the fastest are the most susceptible to damage. They are the cells in the lining of the digestive tract, and in the hair follicles, and the bone marrow cells that make blood cells.

Tolerance to a particular drug or combination of drugs varies with the individual. One person may experience major toxicity while another is minimally affected. I do not like to overemphasize the possibility of side effects because I believe that anxiety about discomfort has produced in some of my patients stronger reactions than they might otherwise have had. I am also convinced that other patients experience mild effects because of their relaxed attitude toward chemotherapy. Although at one time the philosophy of medical therapy was that to be effective, a medicine had to make you sick, chemotherapists generally do not find this to be true. There does not appear to be a direct correlation between the degree of discomfort from drug treatment and the degree of medical effectiveness. The most toxic therapy may be inefficient, while the most favorable results may be obtained when minimal side effects are present.

When side effects do occur, I try to alter a therapy or the method or time of application if this will ease the discomfort of undergoing treatment or help the patient coordinate treatment with his other commitments. For example, working people can often be put on a program that does not interfere with their work schedules. A person with cancer may receive his therapy just before the weekend so that any side effects will have worn off by Monday. Mort Segal (Chapter 5) switched from a morning to an evening chemotherapy program so that he would experience any side effects at home rather than in the office. Joan Stansfield's (Chapter 6) chemotherapy drug content was altered so she could continue to run her household and fulfill her job obligations. The aim is always to keep a patient functioning as fully as possible.

Chemotherapeutic drugs may be administered orally, intramuscularly, or intravenously. Single or multiple drugs may also be infused directly into certain organs, such as the liver, where the disease predominates. The necessity for a weekly office or hospital visit can often be eliminated when chemotherapy is given orally. But when such patient independence is possible, there is still a need for periodic office visits for blood counts and blood chemistry analyses to check on the amount of oral chemotherapy that is needed. A more complex chemotherapeutic program may require more frequent office visits, often three to five days in a row, for a cycle of therapy followed by a rest period. The method by which therapy is given is determined by the physician in consultation with the patient, as well as by the type and stage of malignancy.

There are several ways of monitoring the body's response to therapy, including blood counts, X-ray tests, special isotope scans, blood chemistry panels of liver or kidney function, and other analyses of general body function. These procedures provide a means of detecting toxicity and reducing side effects, as well as of evaluating the effectiveness of treatment. They also serve as safeguards before continuing with current therapy or proceeding with a new form of therapy.

Progress is continually being made. We know more about the method and frequency of administration of effective drugs; we have devised better combinations of those drugs; and new drugs are constantly being developed.

Many cancers are sensitive to hormones, and hormonal anticancer therapy may be the ideal approach for certain kinds of tumors. Cancer of the prostate, breast, or kidney may be controlled or significantly reduced by adding hormonal medication or by reducing the body's production of a hormone.

Experimental Immunotherapy

The concept of immunotherapy is based on the body's natural defense system, which protects us against a variety of diseases. Although we are less aware of it, the immune system also works to aid our recovery from many illnesses. For many years physicians believed that the immune system was effective only in combating infectious diseases caused by agents such as bacteria and viruses. More recently, scientists have learned that the immune system may play a central role in protecting the body against the development of cancer as well as in combating cancer that has already developed. The latter role is not readily apparent, but there is evidence that in many cancer patients the immune system does function to slow down the rate at which tumors grow and spread. More important, the body's ability to develop an immune reaction to tumor may be a decisive factor in determining which patients are cured of cancer by conventional therapy such as surgery, radiation, or drugs.

The immediate goal of research in cancer immunology is to develop new methods to harness and enhance the body's natural tendency to defend itself against malignant tumors. If this can be accomplished, medicine will have a new and powerful weapon to add to the arsenal of anticancer treatments.

Of all the experimental possibilities on the horizon, immunotherapy seems to have the greatest promise of becoming a new dimension in cancer treatment. But it is still very much in its infancy. Although some trials of immunotherapy in humans are in progress, an enormous amount of research remains to be done before these theories can be widely applied to cancer patients.

ANXIETY AND THE ONGOING CONTRACT

In accordance with the terms of the "unwritten contract," I try not to make any medical decisions without taking into consideration the emotional needs of a patient. The more we talk about his family, work, religious views, hobbies, moods, and general life style, the more I learn about what those needs are. At the same time I have to tell him that our choice of a therapy, or a combination of therapies, may be limited at any given time by his type of cancer and its stage of development.

I describe the risks, side effects, and anticipated results of the appropriate therapies, so that there will be no unnecessary shocks in the present or the future. I also explain that it is not uncommon to change from one mode of therapy to another, to alter the dosage or content of a therapy, or even to cease therapy altogether for a time. Such moves should not be misconstrued as a failure of therapy or a progression of disease.

Many patients are overconcerned when changes are made. Others spend their time worrying about the side effects or the effectiveness of their current drug. These are the kinds of anxieties that can be alleviated by a physician during regular office visits. Many of my patients continue to use the "shopping list" method that I suggested in our first talks. A person can be so anxious during an office visit, so fearful of receiving a poor medical report, that he forgets other troubling thoughts and questions that have arisen since his last visit. The "shopping list" reminds him of these concerns and discussion of them relieves him of many anxieties. Having a list of questions at hand also makes the most efficient use of the often limited time of an office visit.

When a particular treatment ceases to be effective, a patient may interpret the withdrawal of that treatment as a signal of imminent death. Such a patient needs to be reassured that there are other methods, or combinations of methods, that may succeed. I was told by one of my patients that I sometimes sound like a sorcerer with a magical bag of tricks, an indefinite number of therapies. Yet it is amazing how often a person who has been successfully treated on a given program and has subsequently relapsed can achieve another remission with a change in therapy. I am not saying that just because a patient accepts treatment, success is guaranteed. We all know there are limits to the possibilities of therapy. The overall cure rate attests to that. But a patient will never know what might have happened unless he is willing to try another therapy, assume the risks, and undergo assessment of the results. This is the practical approach to the treatment of cancer.

It is the job of an oncologist to know what is current and available with regard to cancer therapy, as well as what may be forthcoming from cancer research, so he can send his patients to specialized centers for treatment unavailable elsewhere. Despite assurances that they are receiving the most up-to-date and effective treatment known, some patients are so terrified that they will not accept standard therapy. This pattern is seen most frequently in patients who have been told that currently available therapy holds little promise of curing their disease (but

may offer great benefit in controlling its rate of growth). Unable to accept the fact that modern medicine cannot effect a cure, they compromise much of their remaining life by running in desperation to distant
clinics or other countries in search of a new treatment or a miracle cure.

One patient who came to me for consultation and therapy had previously traveled to both Germany and Mexico with her husband because they had been unwilling to accept the therapy recommended at a
major university cancer center in California. Instead, she tried and still
takes at least twenty different types of vitamins, plus carrot juice, various enzymes, and Laetrile.* I recommended certain alternative medical therapies to this couple, but they were unable to make a choice.
Finally, because valuable time was passing, I said to them, "There is no
sense in my discussing this with you any further until you are willing to
come to a decision. If you want me to decide for you, I'll be happy to
do so. You have two choices at this time: surgery plus radiotherapy or,
should you not want surgery, radiotherapy plus medical therapy—
hormones and/or chemotherapy. I've explained the pros and cons of
both approaches, and although I have a preference, I am not absolutely
certain which is the better treatment. That can be assessed only after a
therapy has been tried and the results graded. If you don't wish to try
either one because of your own fears, that's your business. As far as
I'm concerned, I'll wait to hear from you." This may sound like a tough
approach after my description of the benefits of a reciprocal exchange
between patient and physician, but a decision had to be made. Subsequently, it was made, and it resulted in a dramatic medical improvement with radiotherapy and chemotherapy.

Another patient, Louise Milner, told me she had decided to take a
two-week vacation in Hawaii when she was actually darting off to
Tijuana for Laetrile treatments. The unfortunate results of her flight
are described in Chapter 7.

Panic and flight are one kind of response. There are other reactions
for which I must be watchful. The most gallant among us may begin to
lose his will and feel increasingly fearful after a long period of physical
distress. A woman who had been cheerful under the most trying conditions became bitter and morose after repeated nausea during chemotherapy. A man who had fought in two wars, been wounded several
times, and endured fifteen months of bone cancer without complaint,
was suddenly unable to discuss his case without falling asleep. I try to
deal with these changes by altering medication, by visiting a patient
more frequently to talk with him about his problems and feelings, and
by any other method I can think of that seems appropriate. Obviously

* Laetrile and other quack cures are discussed in the Conclusion.

some problems are resolvable while others are chronic, with no satisfactory solution.

Anxiety does not always originate in a patient's concern with the medical aspects of his cancer. Sometimes it is related to the ordinary pressures of life—the fear of losing a job, or a misunderstanding with a relative or a friend—and compounded by having to cope with cancer. One of my patients holds a responsible, demanding job that could be jeopardized by the limitations on her energy resulting from her cancer and the therapy required. Her teenage children are always in trouble, and her former husband is unable to help emotionally or even to take care of the children when she is hospitalized. As a result of all these worries, she continued to be depressed even after she obtained a remission from anemia and advanced involvement of the liver and bone from breast cancer. However, because she shared her concerns with me, I was able to offer her extra emotional support.

Since it is not always possible to tell solely from office visits what extra burdens a patient must endure in addition to his cancer, I try, if requested, to make a house call early in a relationship. A very well-dressed patient may actually live in minimal circumstances or suffer from tension caused by another family member. One of my patients, a young man with lung cancer, became desperately ill one evening and finally telephoned me. I found him in a rooming house in a deteriorating part of town. He lived in one small room and shared a bathroom at the end of the hall with several other people. When he suffered side effects from radiation, he had to depend on the manager of the rooming house to bring him his meals. He had been too proud to ask for help, but, having discovered his true situation, I was able to mobilize nursing care and other assistance. In the home of another patient I found that life was organized around a senile grandparent to the extent that my patient, who had enough problems of her own, could not leave the house without getting a baby-sitter.

I envisage the role of a physician as an adviser and friend and in this capacity try to help patients plan new approaches. This sometimes involves discussions of how a patient's illness, or the knowledge of his eventual death, is affecting each member of his family. Sometimes, too, when making a will or arranging other personal affairs becomes for the patient an unwelcome acknowledgment that his illness is terminal, I try to encourage him to act for the protection of his family.

I feel that I should become involved in such matters only when a patient indicates receptivity. But at the same time, when it seems to me there is a potential future problem due to a lack of planning, I look for a way to bring this to a patient's attention. I may then be able to provide the proper assistance by introducing my patient to a social worker, an attorney, or some other qualified person. I recently had a patient, Joan (Chapter 6), with terminal cancer, who had little money and was the sole support of a very young child. Joan and I arranged for guardianship of the child by a young married relative well in advance of Joan's death. The assurance that her daughter would grow up in happy circumstances relieved her greatest anxiety.

Listening and talking, an atmosphere of openness and candor, are the means by which an enduring, supportive relationship is developed. If a patient will share his emotional, financial, and other concerns with his physician, he may find unexpected and welcome interest and help. What a patient tells me guides me in each decision regarding the treatment of his cancer and his general well-being; what I tell him —the knowledge of his disease and its treatment, present and future—reduces his anxiety and frees him to direct his thoughts toward life.

But to make such a relationship a reality, a patient must have the wisdom to know his needs and the courage to articulate them to his physician. This is his obligation in a good relationship. Then, if he does speak out and receives no emotional support, he should discuss his frustration with his doctor and suggest the possibility of participating in a supporting program or seeking psychiatric help (see Chapter 16).

REMISSION AND CURE: THE NEED FOR FOLLOW-UP

Most patients who improve on therapy become converts and need only minimal encouragement to sustain their determination as they continue to undergo treatment. Others are reluctant to continue. They may have found that the side effects, even when minimal, are more than they can tolerate. Or they may have undergone surgery, radiotherapy, and medical therapy, reached an improved status, and decided they have endured enough. When such patients announce that they would like to reduce treatments or eliminate them altogether, I must be very convincing if I am to keep them on therapy and thus maintain their stable status.

For instance, an executive who underwent four intensive courses of chemotherapy, combined with immunotherapy, was elated during a period of remission. We warned him we would have to observe his condition closely. Now we suspect a recurrence and he insists that treatment be kept to a minimum. This is, of course, his prerogative.

In regard to follow-up in general, there are some malignancies that need not be treated immediately and a few that need never be treated. The fact that a person has cancer does not necessarily mean he needs instant treatment. Some chronic leukemia patients, with active but not progressive disease, are merely kept under close observation. But whatever the situation, the condition of all past or present cancer patients should be closely monitored over the years, and patients should be well informed about the prospects for recurrence of their cancer. With this knowledge they will be more likely to take the preventive measures that may once again save or prolong their lives.

3 · When Cancer Is Terminal

Death is a part of life. We all must die sometime—we don't know when. Yet we persist in thinking of death as something that happens to other people. We do not accept our mortality until a crisis occurs, and one such crisis, all too frequent in our time, is a diagnosis of cancer. Such a crisis forces us to contemplate nonbeing, to attempt a reconciliation with the fact of impending death. We may fight, bargain, and connive to gain more time, but life is elusive as well as precious. It may be snuffed out at a moment's notice or drain away slowly with disease or old age. And although physicians fight to preserve life at almost any cost in time, money, or effort, we also know a day will come when the time is right to let a patient go.

In partnership with his physician, a cancer patient faces many difficult issues. Throughout treatment he shares in medical decisions, and if his cancer becomes progressively worse, he will at some point discuss with his physician how he wants his death handled. He will tell him where he prefers to spend his last days and what he wants in terms of medical support. He may also tell him what funeral arrangements he wants. The only thing a patient cannot dictate is when he will die, for there are no yardsticks to measure that delicate, highly individual time. Often I have seen a patient and thought that this was his time, only to find him so improved in the next few days that he returned home a week later. That is why I no longer feel that I or anyone else has the ability to predict when another person will die. I prefer to withhold judgment, visit a patient frequently, and continually reassess his condition.

The medical aspects of the terminal phase of his disease are of deep concern to a patient. When should anticancer therapy be stopped? Will his pain be controlled? My general rule is to administer therapy as long as a patient responds well and has the potential for a reasonably good quality of life. But when all feasible therapies have been administered and a patient shows signs of rapid deterioration, the continuation of therapy can cause more discomfort than the cancer. From that time I recommend surgery, radiotherapy, or chemotherapy only as a means of relieving pain. But if a patient's condition should once again stabilize after the withdrawal of active therapy and if it should appear that he could still gain some good time, I would immediately reinstitute active therapy. The decision to cease anticancer treatment is never irrevocable, and often the desire to live will push a patient to try for another remission, or even a few more days of life.

There is an effective therapy to combat any degree of discomfort or pain. I find the most effective procedure is simply to correlate the medication with the complaint. If a patient is nauseated, I give him antinausea medicine. If he is unable to sleep, I prescribe sedatives—barbiturate or nonbarbiturate, depending on his tolerance. And if he has pain, I use an appropriate analgesic or narcotic, as often as needed. The drugs can be administered in pill form, as a suppository, or by injection. A few patients even learn to administer their own shots, as a diabetic does, under medical supervision. Addiction is not a concern when a person has advanced cancer. Moreover, most patients report a tendency to use fewer drugs when they know drugs are readily available if needed. The need for narcotics is alleviated by a satisfactory therapeutic response (surgery, radiation therapy, or chemotherapy) or by other modalities (acupuncture, or nerve blocks by electrical, chemical, or surgical means).

Most people would prefer to be at home when they are sick, especially if they know they have a terminal illness. Any other arrangements will necessarily seem less warm and personal. However, not every household can easily accommodate a patient who needs round-the-clock care. The other family members may be working, or they may be physically unable to carry out some of the more strenuous nursing duties, such as turning the patient or helping him to the bathroom. A patient cared for at home does not have access to the complicated equipment and trained personnel available in a hospital.

Whatever the advantages of a hospital, it is often considered a place of no return, and readmittance can be even more frightening than admittance. People ask if they are going to die or whether they will ever return home. Therefore, just in terms of psychological uplift, it is important that a patient be sent home at the earliest conceivable time.

Extra help is available to solve some problems of home care. Social service agencies, paramedical people such as licensed vocational nurses and nurse's aides, and civic and professional groups such as the American Cancer Society—all offer support. The Cancer Society is often able to provide hospital beds, walkers, bedside toilets, and other equipment, and in certain cities it helps defray the cost of X rays and drugs, and helps arrange transportation to and from treatment (see Chapter 16).

The advantages of going home vary from patient to patient. One of my patients was in the terminal stages of disease when she asked to go home. She could barely walk, had lost her appetite, and required intravenous feeding. Her weight loss exceeded fifty pounds. To carry out her wish we requested help from the American Cancer Society, which provided a walker and a wheelchair and arranged for nursing care at home. The move was made, and the resulting emotional lift contributed to a few extra, rewarding days of life.

But at other times my judgment has been wrong. I have sent a patient home when his family was not prepared to accept the burden or to fulfill his needs and have later been told how destructive the experience was for the patient as well as the family. The stress of prolonged illness often creates unresolvable problems. Other members of the family need to continue with their daily activities, yet they may feel guilty for doing so. A patient may simultaneously feel guilty for being a burden and resentful that he is not receiving sufficient attention and sympathy.

Today more people die in nursing homes and hospitals than at home. Dying in this manner, separated from familiar sights and sounds, can be a doubly lonely ordeal, increasing natural feelings of isolation and abandonment. But if one had to choose between a hospital and a nursing home, I would recommend the former. Nursing homes are frequently run strictly for financial gain and may not have the more elaborate facilities of a regular hospital. Many of these homes will need to be upgraded before they can provide the proper warmth and dignity for anyone, especially for the dying.

An ideal of care in this area is St. Christopher's Hospice, in London, founded by Dr. Cicely Saunders in 1967 as a research, treatment, and teaching facility devoted to meeting the needs of the dying and the long-term sick. Its aims are both control of physical pain and understanding of the emotional and spiritual problems of patients and their families. Dr. Saunders wants her patients to live until they die. The atmosphere is informal, the building designed for maximum openness, space, and light. Families are encouraged to visit at any hour of the day; the staff becomes as friendly with them as with the patients. Children are welcome visitors, and there is a day-care center for the staff's children. Dr. Saunders describes St. Christopher's as offering "intensive personal care," and she feels that it is what staff members do beyond their strictly medical duties that counts most.

Dr. Saunders believes that constant pain needs constant control, so drugs are given regularly rather than when the need arises. This reassures a patient that he will not suffer and forestalls the fear and anxiety that can intensify pain. The goal is to be free of pain, but alert. Drugs are usually given orally rather than by injection, to increase a patient's feelings of independence and to make it easier for him to go home for weekends or longer. The number of patients who are in their own homes at any given time equals the number of patients in the hospice. On the other hand, the hospice has a wing for elderly people, who may live there for years.

For dying patients, St. Christopher's provides the opportunity for them and their families to say a loving good-by, and this is what families will remember: a time of sadness but not of depression, when the person dear to them received affection and physical relief. Similar hospices are now being founded in the United States.

As the final days approach for a patient, I continue to base my decisions on my medical knowledge and my patient's needs and preferences. Our contract is still in effect. I am always ready to be candid. I consider it necessary to reassess each day exactly how much a person really wants to hear. A patient may subtly indicate that he prefers a period of reticence between us concerning the gravity of his situation. For instance, I remember a woman who was in the terminal phase of her disease. She had been through the trials of all the standard and experimental anticancer therapies, and she knew how poor her prospects were. In the past she and I, with her family, had held many frank discussions concerning her progress. Nevertheless, she said to me, "Am I going to die now?" She followed this with, "I know I have cancer, I know it's really bad, I want you to tell me but please don't tell me." The sentence was uninterrupted. There was no pause in her speech.

With whom do you level, and how do you level? I replied, "No. Your gynecologist says the tumor has receded. Your weakness is due to your therapy and to not eating." Misleading? Yes, but she did not ask the definitive question. I am certain she knew the real answer, and on a subsequent visit when her spirits were improved, I knew I had been right to reply as I had because it fulfilled her emotional need of the moment and assured her of my continuing support.

At other times I may postpone giving a patient a candid appraisal of his medical status. Discomfort and pain from progressive disease or the side effects of a drug can affect a person's ability to accept bad news. A depressed patient may interpret any pessimistic statement as a prognosis of imminent death, so I see no sense in making him feel worse by telling him his X rays show progressive disease or his blood counts are more abnormal than yesterday.

Most people know when they are dying and are sensitive to the suffering of those around them, concerned over the emotional stress they are causing the people close to them. Yet sometimes when they express a desire for peace, they are made to feel guilty by relatives who prefer to keep them alive under any conditions. To resolve in advance the possibility of such a conflict, many patients make a verbal agreement with their physician or sign a document called a Living Will (see Appendix III, that states their request not to be kept alive by artificial means or heroic measures when there is no reasonable expectation of recovery.

For some patients there is a preterminal phase that involves a slow descent into a coma. At this time a patient is still alert enough to take comfort in talking with his family or the medical staff, and anything or anyone especially dear to him should be made available. He may want to spend time with a particular relative, friend, child, or even a pet.

However, I must repeat that there are no prophets or prognosticators among physicians who are capable of deciding when a person is going to die. We have only clinical judgment as to the time remaining for any patient. Moreover, no one can prejudge the value of extra days or hours. Some time ago a patient of mine was dying, with marked jaundice, of a massive malignancy that was obstructing his liver. Not wanting him to suffer any longer, I left a verbal order with the interns and the resident that when he died no resuscitative efforts should be employed. About half an hour later the patient had a cardiac arrest. Both the interns and the resident were not in the room, and the nursing staff had changed for the morning shift; the nurse naturally ordered the cardiac resuscitative unit, and the patient was revived. He lived another forty-eight hours, and in that time several relatives arrived from the Midwest and were able to visit with him. In addition, a brother from whom he had been estranged for twenty years flew to San Francisco, and they were reunited. He also had warm, emotionally satisfying talks with his wife and children about their life together.

Another patient, at a hospital where I consulted, was on a ward with twelve others. Often a patient who is close to death is removed to a private room to prevent emotional disturbance among the other patients when he dies, and to provide privacy and convenience for his family and friends, who can then visit him around the clock. This patient was taken to a private room and visited by a priest, but the patient told him emphatically that he did not wish to receive the last rites,* that he wanted to return to the ward. He knew that as long as he was in a private room he was a candidate for death and he did not feel this was his time. He was returned to the ward, where he had some

---

* This sacrament is now called the Sacrament of the Sick.

temporary improvement before dying. He had adjusted to living with cancer over many years, but he needed more time to reconcile himself to dying.

When a patient goes into a final state of coma, I keep him comfortable. This may require a moderate amount of hydration—intravenous feeding and keeping the mouth moist—as well as frequent turning and skin care. In certain cases I may continue to administer narcotics or sedatives at regular intervals even after he is in a coma, if there appears to be restlessness or pain. This reassures his family that any pain or discomfort is being alleviated.

Death is never easy to accept, no matter what the cause. Family members need special attention throughout the ordeal, but especially in those final days. Help may come from within the family, or from friends, but physicians, nurses, clergy, social workers, and hospital volunteers are also available and ready to listen. I always hope that a family will find solace in the knowledge that its loved one received good medical care and sensitive emotional support, that he lived as long and as well as possible under adverse conditions, and that all possible comfort was provided to ease his dying.

Part II
One Patient's View of the Doctor-Patient Relationship

Part II

4 · Ellen Abbott

I think that doctors can perhaps get some satisfaction, as certainly I as a patient have gotten, in being engaged in the fight. It's us against cancer, and we know we aren't going to win in the end, but, by God, we're going to give it a run for its money. And I find this sort of challenging as a patient.

These are the words of a patient living with a fatal disease, not a dying patient. Ellen Abbott discovered on her forty-third birthday that she had advanced ovarian cancer. From what her family and friends tell me, she had always transmitted a special radiance and joy in living, but she lived the last three years of her life with even more enthusiasm than before her illness. The knowledge that she was under a death sentence heightened her zest for life.

At the time of Ellen's treatment I was holding a series of seminars for residents and interns on the problems and concerns of patients faced with terminal cancer. I asked Ellen if she would attend. I felt that the group would benefit from a comparison of her personal experiences with our professional observations, and also that Ellen, with her keen perceptions and analytical mind, could help us to identify and articulate the special problems confronting cancer patients and physicians. Ellen readily agreed to come and became a permanent participant in the seminars.

I also asked Ellen if she would help counsel other cancer patients less well adjusted than herself. Soon both physicians and patients were seeking her advice. Implicit in all she said was her belief that life should be lived. She was convinced, as I am, that each person with cancer has the potential to remain productive and to enjoy life during most of his illness.

The way Ellen dealt with her own terminal illness is proof that she was able to translate her ideas into action. She was, and will remain, an inspiration to her family and friends, her doctors, and the other patients who had the privilege of knowing her.

I once asked Ellen whether there was anything special she would like to accomplish before she died and she replied that she would like to write a guidebook for other patients, to share with them the positive aspects of her experience with cancer.

I have had a good time of it and I think I could write something that would help others. There are lots of things a patient can do in managing his doctors and family and even his own moods. At the same time a physician has to set the tone in advance for the patient. I'd like to help just some physicians feel, "Gee, I could do this or be that . . ." and also some patients—some in very practical terms and others in a perhaps more philosophical sense—take it easier.

Ellen died before she could write her guidebook, but the following pages contain many of her observations, taken directly from the transcripts of our tape-recorded seminars.

A hundred years ago people grew up on farms. They saw birth and death all the time with the animals. Death was a natural part of life. They saw it as part of the rhythm of life, and one got a larger sense of the seasons, birth, death, life and so on. It's really in the past fifty years in this country and in other industrialized countries that people don't see life and death in the great pattern.

My father was a doctor and so I think that I became realistic at a very young age. I understood that if certain things happened, they were pretty much going to happen. I got this understanding from him, a certain acceptance, so that although like all of us I had never thought I was going to die at all, the minute I heard what had happened to me and how widespread it was, then I knew that nothing was going to change. I don't think you really know if you are going to be afraid or not. I think before I would probably have thought so, but as soon as I knew what was wrong and what was going to happen, I wasn't.

I have no fearful associations with death. I have never thought I was being punished for my sins. I have sinned, I suppose, but I never believed in any sort of cosmic justice or injustice. I never bargained for my life because I didn't think there was anyone who would intervene. I think the universe is neutral. I assume that if you get cancer cells and they spread, the forces of nature are going to go on and you are going to die.

I imagine death as the big sleep. I don't believe in an afterlife; I think it is the end. I know some people despair because of that, but I assume that's the way it is. That's my concept of death and I think that's why I'm not afraid to die—although I want to live as long as I can because I have everything to live for, but that's different from fearing to die.

It helps too that I've always loved life and have no regrets. My father said that he had found that unhappy people were much worse about dying than happy people. They feel they have not lived and they aren't ready to go yet. I don't think that I've lived my life. I thought I'd live to be ninety. But I think that the awareness of not having lived while you can must be frustrating to people. An awful lot of people don't live. They don't enjoy life as they go along and then suddenly it's too late.

Living

Ellen's early reconciliation with death allowed her more freedom to live. Having made this essential adjustment, she had no fear and was able to redirect her energies. When this psychological process of reconciliation does not occur, the fear of death can immobilize a patient.

The fear of cancer can be equally paralyzing, and Ellen recalled her own exposure to the taboos surrounding that word.

I'm convinced that Roosevelt was right when he said that the only thing we have to fear is fear itself, blind unreasoning fear. By fear I don't mean legitimate fear—I mean, cancer's something to fear, but do you know what I mean? You all know that there is associated with cancer, particularly, this strange aura. Why is it so much worse than other things? I am not being a Pollyanna, but there are other terrible diseases.

There's always been a taboo. A generation ago my own mother —just to give you an idea—a doctor's wife—never used the word cancer, until I got it; and then she spoke it because I always said "cancer." You almost had to whisper, "So-and-so has a malignancy." Now why that's a better word, I don't know. My dad would just say "C.A."

During a meeting of the seminar in which these matters were discussed, an intern remarked that he had seldom seen a doctor successfully handle the problem of death. Ellen was appalled.

I don't think it's as fancy a problem as you all think. People have been dying for thousands of years and managed to carry it off pretty well. It isn't so mysterious and arcane that a good physician, a good human being with respect for another human being, cannot somehow convey both his strength and support.

However, Ellen thought the current wave of books and articles about death might provide a rationale for a doctor to avoid meeting his responsibilities to patients. He might be tempted to think that since he was not a psychiatrist, he was not qualified to help a patient face death. Another physician might take as a personal and professional defeat the eventual loss of two out of three patients. His tendency might then be to concentrate on patients whom he could cure, absolving himself of responsibility to his terminal patients with the comforting thought that research will one day provide a cure. In the meantime, many of these patients who were not going to benefit from future research would be walking around half dead, crippled not by cancer but by fear.

Ellen and I therefore felt that physicians should establish realistic goals for the treatment of terminal cancer patients, with victory measured by the number of active years or months gained for each person.

A cancer patient's ability or inability to live fully while undergoing treatment often reflects the way he lived before his cancer was discovered, but Ellen found that a patient-doctor relationship based on candor and trust makes it easier for a patient to concentrate on living.

The physician is the most important person in a terminal patient's life. He may not be the most beloved or valuable, but he has the most telling effect on the kind of life the patient leads. No one— parent, child, husband, lover, or best friend—can take the physician's place. Having had cancer for more than two years, I know what a doctor can mean in liberating one to live actively during the remaining time of one's life.

A doctor should recognize that by his own courage and respect for the patient, he can relieve terror. If he shows confidence that he can remain in control of the disease and the pain, it removes an enormous burden from the patient's life. This is the approach my doctors have taken with me. It was never spoken, but they communicated it in their actions and manner. And it has been a wonderful feeling. Instead of seeing each setback and loss of time as a defeat, we turn it around. Each day, week, and month that we pass—particularly if I am free to enjoy life during that time —is a victory.

If I had not trusted my physicians, I would have spent my time wondering, "Where's it going to go next?" or "Is the pain going to be so bad they won't be able to control it?" Instead I told myself, "That's their problem. I have enough to do handling my family and friends and everybody else, doing all the things I want to do." So I put the responsibility on the doctors. Naturally, I tell them my symptoms and cooperate with them. I do everything they tell me, but basically all of the therapy is up to them; I don't have to worry about it.

If a doctor can add to the quality of life of his patient, if he can let the patient live while he's living, there is no greater gift. Even if he could prolong life or save it, I would be willing to say that perhaps the greater gift is this liberating of a life that he is bound to lose ultimately.

When I left the hospital for the first time I asked Dr. John Kerner, my gynecologist, that question I shouldn't have asked,

"How long?" That was the only time he ever evaded me, and rightly. Because doctors don't know. He evaded me by saying, "Well, the statistics are quite unreliable, and after all, if you're the 1 percent . . ." And then—it's funny, it was the first time I ever thought consciously about any of this—I said, "Now that I think about it, I don't think I would do anything terribly differently if you said six months. I really enjoy life so much the way it is. I would like to go on living pretty much that way." He replied, "I wouldn't put anything off once you start to feel well. The way to live is to live."

The First Meetings Between Patient and Physician

In January 1972, Ellen, my wife, Isadora, and I attended a symposium called Current Concepts in Medical Oncology. One of the speakers was an anthropologist who, like many others there, concentrated on the patient's last days and hours. He suggested that true dying occurred in this final phase of life and that a patient is often abandoned at this most important time. Ellen did not agree with this definition of the "most important time" in the experience of a cancer patient.

I have not gone through the terminal phase yet, but a year ago I believed I was going to die and nearly did. Before the terminal stages, the relationship between patient and physician is formed, and any late efforts to save or correct it are bound to fail. The patient is too consumed by fear and pain to develop a meaningful relationship with anyone at this time.

It is in the earliest meetings, even before the diagnosis, that the tone of the relationship is set. In these encounters, the physician reveals his attitudes toward the disease and the patient. He establishes the foundation of confidence and support on which the patient will later rely. If he shows respect for the patient and his own courage in the face of cancer, he will immediately begin to win the patient's trust. It is important to achieve this before the diagnosis because the physician's manner in presenting the diagnosis and the patient's reaction to it have an enormous effect on the course of the disease.

It happened so quickly that I was completely taken aback and forced to acknowledge what happened. Before the operation I asked my gynecologist to level with me completely. Following surgery, he told me what they had done and what they had not been able to do, and then I knew. I remember I thought, "So." It was resignation. He kept talking, and I cannot recall everything he said, but obviously he was very good in the way he handled me. He was planning radiation therapy. He never pretended that he could save me. He did not say, "You're going to die," but he told me enough so that I knew. Still, he was very positive about therapy. He was not afraid of the disease, and that, along with the respect he showed by being honest, led me to put my confidence in him.

One of the reasons Ellen adjusted so successfully was that Dr. Kerner treated her with sensitivity and respect. Later, while counseling other terminal patients, Ellen often became depressed by stories they told of the unintentional cruelty their primary doctors had shown in telling them about their disease and their prospects for recovery. In many cases the effects of these encounters could not be undone by subsequent supportive efforts of friends, relatives, or physicians.

The nameless, formless fear of cancer and death can be very upsetting to a patient, and this is what is contributed to when a physician is not candid and confident. When the physician is dishonest, the patient thinks, "If my doctor can't tell me, if he can't face it, it must be really terrible. What's the end going to be like?" The patient communicates this fear to his relatives and friends and soon the mood infects everyone. In these circumstances, the patient may refuse to believe anything the doctor tells him and exhaust himself worrying about the progress of the disease.

The physician's demeanor over a good length of time is also important. It isn't just the first interview. It's over and over. It's the whole thing. I think one of the best things that has happened with my doctors is that so often a question is trembling on my lips, and before I can even say it, one of them says, "You realize . . ." or "You know why we're doing so and so . . ." Or sometimes they have anticipated further than that and told me something I would have wanted to know in a day or two.

Pain

A physician must be flexible and adjust treatment according to changes in a patient's physical and mental condition, because fear of pain and of the future may increase as disease progresses. Ellen Abbott was free from excessive anxiety about pain, but she was realistic about its effects. At one time she suffered a severe relapse from an intestinal obstruction. Unable to eat, she weighed seventy-seven pounds instead of her normal weight of one hundred fifteen, and had to have a tube drain her stomach and intestines. It was then that I first met Ellen, having been called in for consultation and to recommend a new chemotherapeutic regime. Almost immediately we developed a good doctor-patient relationship, which was further strengthened when she responded to the medical maneuvers. Her partial intestinal obstruction was reversed; she regained thirty pounds and was able to return to active living.

It is not dying but pain that I fear. I am not haunted by it because I do not think my doctor will let me go through unendurable suffering. But pain can be a terribly dehumanizing and degrading experience. You feel like an animal. All you think about is the pain and how to get out of it. There are no higher thoughts, no philosophy, no religion, or anything else. Even your nearest and dearest do not mean much to you. When I felt very sick, the only human thing I did was think about the millions of people in the world who are in agony without a bit of comfort; the napalm and the people in Vietnam without doctors. I thought, "My God, what that must be. Alone, without anyone, lying in a ditch." That hit me. No comfort and nobody to ease them. And here I was with people hovering, offering help and giving help.

I had Demerol when I was so sick last winter, in great pain, and Ernie showed me how to "shoot it" or whatever you do. Sometimes I have terrific pain, but right now, I feel just great. I have narcotics—dolophine, percodan, codeine, and things like that. But I don't have any temptation to take them except when I really need them, and usually I don't need them. There hasn't been any temptation to abuse drugs.

But at that time (last winter) I really thought I was going to die, although I never completely gave up hope. And it was a slow recovery. I was in bed for five to six months. Although part of it was very rough, I thought—and this was again partly because of the confidence that had been established with my doctors—that they weren't asking me to go through all that for nothing. I think they probably thought that the chances were very poor of my coming through that crisis, but that on the other hand, if I did, I would have a really good remission, which I have had. I never thought they were saving me just to remain in that state all the time.

At one of the meetings of the seminar an intern asked Ellen whether she would mind discussing her feelings about suicide.

I'd be glad to talk about it. My intellectual feeling is that everybody has a right to his life. I can conceive intellectually of coming to that moment of despair but I'm not yet able to conceive of it emotionally because, as you can see, I'm enjoying myself so much that I want to go on as long as I can.

I'm in the same position you are in. All of you said that when you think about death, it's still a little abstract to you. So although I believe absolutely intellectually that I have the right to take my life when it gets to the point where it's too rough, when the outlay is too great and the pain and the trouble—frankly, emotionally, it's hard to imagine that time.

But if I knew there was never going to be another fairly good remission, where there was going to be any good time, then I would prefer not to have to do it myself. I would say to Ernie or to John, "Let me go." I have that faith in both my doctors.

Ellen panicked only once, when she had a pulmonary embolus, a blood clot in the lungs. She required oxygen and had great difficulty in breathing. There was a tube in her chest to remove collected fluid, and an intravenous tube feeding fluid support and anticoagulants into her vein. At the height of the episode she became panicky. She was cyanotic —ashen colored—gasping for breath as if she were drowning. It was enough to terrify the most resolute person. Her fear lasted less than a day, although her medical crisis continued for three days. Later she was remorseful and apologized for not being as noble as she had wanted to be. "It's not the way I want to die," she said. Ellen had repeatedly said she was not afraid of death and had talked to patients about how to maintain their composure. Now she thought she was a failure and felt she had let down her friends, her doctor, and herself. I tried to convince her that her reactions were normal and asked her if she did not feel she had a right to respond like anyone else, but she was not very forgiving of herself.

Family and Friends

Ellen's high personal standards sometimes led to depression of another kind. She knew that the will to live was important, and she wanted to feel she was making the maximum effort at all times. Occasionally, when she was unable to accomplish as much as she had planned, she would be cheered when I told her that it was her disease, not herself, that was limiting her desire and capacity for achievement. Such depressions were infrequent. Ellen found, on the contrary, that physical activity was all that was reduced. Every other sense and feeling expanded and flourished because of her altered circumstances.

Disease rearranges your values and you cast off things. You do not put up with a lot of stuff in your own self. You reduce the trivia to a minimum. You simplify life, as Thoreau said, when you are under a death warrant.

There is nothing to be afraid of any more when you know you are going to die. It is liberating, very liberating. All the lies are dropped and it cleans up your life. Then everything becomes more poignant, more vivid, the people you love and the people you do not. Relationships become better. You are more aware of the love you feel on both sides, if you know that someone is not going to be there forever. But I also think it's because of the added candor, that you are sharing something together with people who love you.

I always enjoyed life, but I've learned to love it more now. Beauty and music, everything is more poignant. Colors are more vivid. The people I love appear more alive. In a way, my life seems in a rut because I cannot do as much, and I do not feel well part of the time. But it is not a rut, because it is so intense. Everything is heightened, and the awareness is just incredible.

Ellen found that selfishness is essential for survival in the sense that each person has the right to live and die on his own terms. She felt it was too complicated to try to protect people, and she was determined to establish an atmosphere of candor in all her relationships.

You have to tell your family and friends. From the beginning I told people what it was. I said it was the big thing, it was cancer. And I don't mean that I didn't act depressed. I said, "I'm going to have all this treatment and everything, but it was pretty bad and they weren't able to get it all." You have to do this, because no one knows how to treat somebody who has cancer. No one will talk about it unless you do. The patient has to set the tone for his surroundings.

Yet one of the surprising reactions was a combination of denial and solicitude. The two things often come together, which is fascinating. I have friends who were as scared of the word as my mother. They wouldn't even say "cancer." They would call it my "disease" or "illness," or "it" or "that." I would very deliberately say, "Well, with cancer . . ." a number of times, hoping they would pick it up. Some simply would not say it. Others refused to acknowledge there was anything wrong.

Last year, I had a relapse and went down to seventy-seven pounds. I looked terrible. Some of the people who love me best would visit me and say, "You're looking wonderful." Just patent lies, and yet they would never accept that I really was going to die of it ultimately. And on the other hand they would help me lift packages years after I had surgery. You get weird oversolicitude and second-guessing, such as, "You probably wouldn't want to go because you'd get tired." It's as though you're not a person any more. But if a patient is tough enough, he can handle it. Over and over you've got to establish the way you're going to handle it and people usually take their cues.

The good thing is, if you're honest, you get past all that and then there is a normal relationship again. Whereas I think if there is a lot of deception, if you're always lying or trying to cover up pain and fatigue, then people think it's worse than it is. If I don't feel good, I don't try to hide it. In fact, you may be full of IVs and terribly sick and everything, but other people will accept it better if you're obviously accepting it in a sense and don't feel destroyed. Then I think they say, "Oh, that's the way it is."

The Patient Treats Her Physicians

Doctors are human. We are depressed by patients who are cold and bitter. We are invigorated by patients who are friendly and cooperative. In all my practice Ellen was the epitome of the kind of patient who makes you glad you are a physician. I looked forward to her visits, as did she.

It would be inaccurate to portray Ellen as a patient who did not have recurring medical crises with the usual slow periods of recovery. She also had many episodes of weakness and abdominal swelling and pain from the partial intestinal obstruction. It was her courage, equanimity, and faith in meeting each crisis that made her such a valued patient.

In a subtle way Ellen was effectively giving therapy to the medical team by encouraging us to do our best even though we could not cure her. She felt compassion for us. She would even urge us not to feel discouraged when she was ill from the side effects of a particular therapy, or when her condition worsened. For such a patient there even comes a time when he feels sympathy for his doctor because he knows his death will be an emotional crisis for the doctor, who is losing a friend. One day during the period of Ellen's pulmonary embolus her mother told a friend, "You know, the thing that's driving Ellen crazy is what it's doing to Ernie."

In essence, Ellen turned something destructive into a positive thing. She used her experience with cancer to help teach some of her physicians how to help terminal patients. During the first meeting of the seminar, Ellen asked the interns there whether they had felt uncomfortable with her or guarded about expressing themselves at the beginning of the evening.

JIM: I think you could probably tell that there was a tremble in my voice when I started expressing some of my ideas, and that was not just because I was having a conversation with someone I'd never known before. It's the fact that you have cancer and you're dying from it.

ELLEN: Now, can you tell me, is it easier or harder for you, now that you've talked with me?

JIM: Oh, extremely easier.

ELLEN: Isn't it a lot easier to talk, but also to think about it? This isn't why I've done this. That's not why I do it; I do it for my own sake. I'm selfish. But I would still guess it makes it easier, really, on other people, too.

JIM: I was thinking about that while you were talking, when we first came here. And this might be cold, but I was just looking at you as an object, and now I feel so much.

TAYLOR: As a disease, a disease, not a person!

JIM: And now I see you as a human being. And it's very positive.

ELLEN: This is the key . . .

TAYLOR: Personally, the first thing I was struck by was, "This can't be Ellen. This can't be the one Dr. Rosenbaum was talking about."

ELLEN (laughing): She's not sick!

TAYLOR: She looks beautiful.

When Ellen began to fail, I asked her whether she would like to return to the hospital or remain at home. She replied that she hadn't really thought about it, but that she did not have the horror of hospitals that some people have, and had always had good treatment from the staff at Mt. Zion. However, she said she enjoyed being at home in familiar surroundings, where her family could be comfortable and her friends could visit easily.

As it happened, Ellen died quietly at home. Shortly before she died, she told her mother, "I have no bitterness, no resentment. I don't even hate cancer. You shouldn't grieve for one whose life has been full and happy."

Part III
Self-Image

Disease is an assault on a person's self-image. A sense of worth is directly related to what we do, how we feel, and how we interact with others, and there are many ways in which having cancer can affect these vital aspects of self. For instance, when a cancer patient is unable to work as hard as he did before his illness, or has less energy for family activities than he used to, he may have feelings of shame or guilt. If his disease is terminal, his sense of being defective and somehow to blame for his condition may be intensified.

These destructive feelings do not, however, originate entirely with a patient. Healthy people tend, at least subconsciously, to think of a person with a serious disease as lacking in some important way. Such attitudes can result in awkward behavior—avoidance, embarrassment, over-solicitude, a tendency to treat a patient as if he were a child. None of this escapes the patient, who is already feeling sensitive about his condition. To be treated differently now must seem a confirmation of his growing feelings of inadequacy. For these reasons a cancer patient, or any other person with a long-term illness, needs an inner certainty of his continuing worth if he is not to fall prey to the attitude of the healthy toward the sick.

Psychological damage can also result from the effects of cancer surgery. A woman whose breast has been removed, and who may even be cured, may have to go through an additional period of anxiety before reaffirming her sexual attractiveness. Surgery that affects the face or neck—areas visible to the public—can also produce self-consciousness and require a period of readjustment. For a person whose livelihood depends on physical perfection—a model or a dancer, for example—the psychological blow of physical impairment can be doubly severe.

Others, accustomed to playing an active role in business and other matters, feel especially humiliated by the loss of autonomy that may accompany progressive disease. When work and accomplishment are a chief source of pleasure and self-definition, slow physical decline can become unbearable.

Most people meet these psychological endurance tests very well, although occasionally a person whose self-esteem was never very high accepts too readily an image of himself as a helpless patient and abandons himself to a brooding acceptance of his bad luck. Sometimes, conversely, patients will report the emergence of a stronger self-image. They say that before having cancer they often felt hindered in their ability to enjoy themselves, either because of a private fear or neurosis or because of the destructive behavior of someone close to them. The realization that their lives might be cut short made their habitual problems appear trivial and even manageable. I do not mean to imply that these people did not also experience rage, regret, or depression, but the ease with which they began to direct their lives produced a kind of exhilaration, an enhancement of self-esteem.

A cancer patient must struggle against many odds to maintain his equanimity. Some people will be awkward in his presence because the taboos and fears associated with cancer are not going to vanish overnight. At other times a discouraging medical report will disrupt his calm. Another day he may feel that medical treatment is an endless invasion of his sense of dignity and privacy. Each time his equilibrium is shattered, it must be slowly regained. Of course, these dynamics become more complicated when cancer is progressive.

Following are the stories of five patients who spoke particularly of the effects of cancer on their self-image, on their way of thinking about themselves and acting in the world.

5 · Mort Segal

When Mort Segal was shown the first draft of this chapter, he felt it did not fully reflect his feelings about his experience with cancer. Because he was a writer, among other things, he began to rewrite the material. Unfortunately, he completed only the first section, entitled "May 16, 1972." Although I urged him many times to continue writing and he often said he wanted to, he never again picked up the manuscript. I feel that if he had tried to complete the chapter, it would have seemed to him that he was completing his life.

May 16, 1972

I had a call at home in the evening from an insurance man I know. He urged me to see a client of his, Mort Segal by name. He told me that Segal had just come over to see him that evening to discuss his insurance policies. Segal had learned earlier in the day that he had a malignant cancer, one that "might kill him in six to eight weeks." Segal's doctor had assured him that these weeks would be extremely rewarding in terms of his family and friends. I was told that Segal was "distressed," which was hardly surprising.

Segal was forceful and energetic, very much in command. He was forty years old, trained as a lawyer, and the managing partner of a national consulting firm specializing in governmental legislative and administrative reforms, governmental reorganization, and the like. It is a field quite outside my experience.

Segal was married and had two young children. He introduced himself as one who had "never been ill" until this "crazy illness" caught up with him. He was annoyed, perhaps even angry, rather as one might feel over having had one's vacation postponed or cut short at the last minute. He appeared determined, at the very outset, to establish a peer relationship with me in regard to the discussion and, even more, the treatment of his disease. He made it clear that he had no intention of merely acquiescing to treatment, as most patients might when consulting their physicians.

Segal made one other point, in very clear and certain terms. He said he would not agree to any treatment unless he was himself satisfied that the likelihood of its success substantially outweighed its physical and psychological inconveniences. "No fishing expeditions," Segal admonished. This point had reference to any of the four cancer therapies: surgery, chemotherapy, radiotherapy, and immunotherapy.

His rationale was that each such treatment intruded upon his basic dignity and privacy, surgery more than chemotherapy, chemotherapy more than radiotherapy, and so on. For Segal, this was to be his private "battle." In a way, he almost appeared to relish the contest. Interference from the sidelines, such as by me, was not going to be readily tolerated. Segal said that if it were not for his wife and little children, if he were single and alone, he would not tolerate any interference at all. It was clear that he would be a difficult, headstrong patient.

Having established the rules of our relationship, Segal went on to describe the course of his illness from its beginning. As it happened, its beginning went back nearly a year in time. It wasn't neat, nor did it move in a single direction. But then, these things seldom do.

Segal told me that on June 24 of the previous year, 1971, he quite suddenly had a sharp pain in his right chest. At the time, he was between planes at O'Hare Airport, outside Chicago, on his way back from Washington, D.C., to San Francisco. The pain immobilized him, so that he was unable to board his plane. He assumed he was suffering a heart attack, which he informed me was "pretty much in accord with the way I always thought I would go." His condition attracted some attention among others waiting for planes. Segal said he was embarrassed by the attention, and attempted to diminish the importance of his condition. Nonetheless, he must have looked fairly bad, and finally he allowed himself to be escorted to the airport's first-aid station. His chest pain became progressively more excruciating.

After several hours of waiting at the airport's first-aid station, Segal agreed to go to a nearby hospital. He refused, however, to sit in the wheelchair provided by the attendants who arrived in an ambulance, and refused to ride in the back of the ambulance as well, sitting up front instead. Numerous X rays were taken at the hospital. Meanwhile, the excruciating pain slowly subsided. After several demeaning hours of waiting, the physician in charge announced triumphantly that Segal was suffering from constipation. Having missed the last direct flight to San Francisco, he left the hospital by taxi and checked into a nearby hotel. Segal called his wife and merely said that he had missed the last plane. He told her he would catch the first plane out of Chicago the next morning.

Upon Segal's return to San Francisco, he underwent a number of tests. The pain had completely disappeared during the course of the night in Chicago. This new battery of tests failed to show any problems. It was finally concluded that Segal might have passed a kidney stone. In any case, the incident was consigned to the nether region of medical science, where symptoms wait to be forgotten or recur.

After the June 24 incident, but quite apart from it, Segal decided to take a year's leave of absence from his firm and move to the south of France. His understanding with his partners covered the possibility that he might simply decide to stay there indefinitely. He and his family were due to leave for Paris on October 1. Their house was accordingly rented, the car sold, and furniture readied for storage.

On September 20, however, Segal experienced a second seizure, this time in the midst of an important business meeting. He collapsed and was taken by ambulance to a San Francisco hospital. He arrived with "no perceptible signs of life." An X ray revealed total opacity of the right lung. A needle was introduced and pure blood was taken. His perivascular status remained precarious for several hours, but finally stabilized enough to permit exploratory thoracic surgery. During the brief time when Segal regained consciousness before surgery, he expressed distress at his passivity in relation to the physicians and others surrounding him. He said he wasn't accustomed to playing a passive role and found it demeaning, if not emasculating. Before being taken in for surgery, he suggested that the surgeon perform a vasectomy he had long planned but had been equally long in postponing.

Segal spent nine hours in the operating room. On three different occasions it looked as if he would die. He received twenty-one pints of blood, and the lower lobe of his right lung was removed. The surgeon also removed a small, exceedingly rare carcinoid-like tumor. The diagnosis was that it was basically benign, although the area ought to be watched. A hospital convalescence of four to six weeks was anticipated, but Segal managed to have himself released within seven days. He worked intermittently at his office for several more weeks, and at the end of October boarded a plane for France with his family.

By the end of April 1972, only six months after leaving San Francisco, the Segals became thoroughly bored with their leisurely life in France. Accordingly, Segal alone flew back to San Francisco, rented an apartment for his family, who would follow within a month, and went back to work at his old desk in his consulting firm. With some reluctance, he decided that the bucolic life in France could not be his life, and that however much he wanted to be a "family man," close to his wife and children, he could not. He was soon flying around the country, rushing from New York to Honolulu, attending meetings and giving consultations.

During his first month back he discovered that a small lump had developed under the thoracic scar tissue of his right chest wall. His physician diagnosed it as a subcutaneous cyst. Shortly thereafter he had it excised one afternoon in his surgeon's office, under a local anesthetic. The surgeon remarked laconically that the subcutaneous cyst was, in fact, a tumor, and that its development was probably attributable to some cell contamination which remained from the original surgery the previous September.

The biopsy of the tumor, done at another hospital from Segal's original operation, showed that it was not the same type as the original tumor, and that, moreover, it was a rare malignancy—a sarcoma. Further comparison of the slides showed that, in fact, both tumors were the same, which is to say that the original biopsy diagnosis had been incorrect. Segal was informed that he had a highly malignant, rare tumor of the blood vessel lining, called hemangiopericytoma. His hemangiopericytoma proved to be the ninth such tumor, in that presentation, known anywhere in the world. It was at that point that Segal's surgeon informed him that the tumor "might kill" him "in six to eight weeks." That evening Segal called his insurance man, who in turn called me.

Late October 1972

Segal refused all treatment for the four months following his diagnosis, preferring to enjoy the short time he was told remained to him. During that time and from then on, my role in his case was that of a consulting physician, working closely with Dr. Herman A. Schwartz, head of oncology at Kaiser Hospital, which was a participant in Segal's health-insurance plan. I explained to Segal that the surgeon's figure was based on an estimate and that the outcome of any one case could not be determined by average statistics, especially when they were based on a sample of only eight other cases. Each case, whether cardiac or cancer, must be considered individually. Segal's reply was always, "If I'm going to die, I want to do it my way."

However, when Segal found he was still alive in mid-October, he became interested in consultations about chemotherapy. (His tumor was not operable for cure at that time, and it was not considered primarily radiosensitive.) He told me that during the six weeks following his prognosis he had leaped from bed each morning ready to do battle with death and that each evening he had had the satisfaction of having won. When the six weeks passed and he was still functioning and well, he felt even more exhilarated, believing that by an act of will he had succeeded in defeating cancer and death.

Although Segal had never been ill himself, he knew what prolonged disease could do to a person's resolve to die with dignity and grace. His father had contracted Parkinson's disease fifteen years before and at the time was adamant about wishing to live only as long as he could take care of himself. His decline was imperceptibly slow, and as the years passed and his debility increased, he abandoned his resolve. Although totally incapacitated, he clung to life. This experience left an indelible impression on Segal and was certainly an important reason for his reluctance to accept treatment.

Another reason, certainly, was that illness is humiliating because a person has to depend on the decisions of others for treatment of a disease he does not completely understand. A doctor tells a patient that certain physical manifestations have been detected and that a particular treatment may be effective in restoring his health. The patient must then trust his physician. Segal was not used to being in this relationship to someone else. He saw his life in terms of his own will.

> Basically I really like the kind of person I've made myself become, and that's what it's all about—whether my will prevails over my doctors', whether I will control the course of my illness and its effects on me. I can do that in a variety of ways, one of which is the decision whether to take treatment or not. It is my intention to die with dignity, not to waste away. I'm not going to go down the tube slowly. The trick is to figure out when that may happen and to act before you lose the option.

We had many sessions, with questions and more questions. Segal played the role of defense attorney and was also his own client. I reminded him of the adage that a lawyer who conducts his own defense has a fool for a client. I could reason with Segal, but I always felt I was losing, and I was surprised to find I had finally won his agreement to try to fight his cancer. Presumably he had come to see me because he had decided to take therapy but he needed to have these arguments first, partly to let me know he was not "turning himself over to me." To assuage his last vestiges of doubt, I sent him to the M. D. Anderson Hospital in Houston for consultation. The concurrence of those doctors with a plan for chemotherapy made Segal receptive to treatment, although he always managed to add another "condition." When he yielded on one issue, he wanted compromise on another.

With the understanding that we didn't know how such a rare tumor would respond to drugs, Dr. Schwartz instituted a four-drug chemotherapy program, to be administered by the physicians at Kaiser Hospital.

Late November 1972

Segal received injections five mornings a week every three weeks and suffered side effects of nausea, vomiting, hair loss, and fatigue. But once he had made the decision to try the program, his determination to see it through prevailed.

The dosage in his daily injections was reduced but the vomiting continued, causing physical discomfort as well as embarrassment. The nausea began just as Segal arrived at work after his morning injection, and it came in unpredictable waves. If he got an attack while in a meeting or on the telephone, he had to excuse himself and rush to the bathroom, where he would vomit for several minutes. These attacks were usually dry heaves and the sound reverberated through the office. He began keeping a bowl in his office, eliminating the dash to the bathroom. Although Segal described these maneuvers with his customary humor, the procedure obviously offended his sense of privacy. We changed the chemotherapy schedule, and his physicians began to administer injections in the evening so he could work uninterrupted during the day.

Chemotherapy also disrupted Segal's travel schedule. He was so uncomfortable during the five days he received injections that he stayed close to home and then tried to squeeze three weeks of travel into two. The vomiting and fatigue reduced his efficiency to such an extent that he often worked all night at the office, returning home around 5:00 A.M. for a few hours of sleep before returning to the office. He was determined to maintain his former level of productivity, which in the past had involved working eighty to ninety hours a week and traveling almost a quarter of a million miles a year.

December 18, 1972

X rays showed changes in Segal's lungs; his disease had returned; which meant that we had to consider surgery. A resection could possibly have reduced the size of the tumor, making it easier to control the residual tumor with chemotherapy and perhaps immunotherapy.

But Segal was against surgery. He recalled with some chagrin that after his first operation he accidentally saw his medical folder, which contained the comment "Shows considerable anxiety about dying." Questioned by Segal, his physician told him, "You were very anxious about dying before the operation; you asked if you were going to die." Segal then asked me whether this had been intellectual curiosity or fear. "Fear. Not weeping, but real fear," I said. This surprised Segal, for fear had no place in his self-image. "My concept of dignity is not to weep when I am dying." The incident had other ramifications—an intrusion on privacy, the humiliation of dependence on the decisions of others, a feeling of anxiety such as some people feel when another person is driving the car.

Segal was determined not to let false hope interfere with his reason, creating the paradox that his emotions in the form of his desire for independence were leading him to make unsound decisions. He refused to yield to my medical experience.

I felt somewhat ambiguous on that point, however, because I believe a patient should participate as much as possible in decisions concerning his treatment. But Segal's need for authority outweighed his knowledge, a fact that caused him some conflict.

This is the first time that I've been in a position where, technically, someone knows significantly more than I do. I have to believe you aren't trumping up enthusiasm to talk me into one more treatment.

The members of the Tumor Board at Segal's hospital were to recommend whether surgery should be performed. Segal remained opposed to an operation but held hours of discussions with his wife, close friends, and doctors. I feel that patients often obtain better medical results when they encourage their physicians to act positively, so I was pleased when Segal eventually acquiesced to surgery.

Late January 1973

On the day Segal was scheduled to enter the hospital, the members of the Tumor Board decided his tumor was too advanced to be treated surgically. Segal's wife, Janet, describes this decision as an enormous letdown for Segal, after he had prepared himself psychologically for the operation. "It was the most painful period for Mort. He kept doing, saying, laughing, joking, directing, inspiring, enraging, but he knew he wasn't going to win the war he cared most about."

Early March 1973

We continued with a program of chemotherapy, but Segal resented the loss of time involved in going for treatment and the interruption in his travel schedule, although he now dismissed the side effects as "inconvenient." I asked him if having cancer had made him change the way he lives.

I don't put things off now, but I never did. I never worried about quitting a job or dropping everything and going off to live in France. Janet and I haven't let ourselves be constrained by finances or the children. People ask me why I don't take a vacation or do something I've always wanted to do. I've always done what I wanted, and what I want to do now is work. My regret in dying isn't for the things I haven't done but for the time I won't have to do more. By rights I should have another fifteen or twenty good years, and now they're gone. You know, I used to kid myself that

I never got to spend time with my family because I had to work so hard, but after the six months in France I realized that I work all the time because I like it. If you feel good about yourself, if you are doing what you want to do, you don't change your life just because you're sick.

June 22, 1973

The tumor in Segal's right chest grew steadily and appeared to be invading his liver. We decided to discontinue chemotherapy because there had been no improvement after six sequences of drugs; and despite Segal's light dismissal of the side effects as little more than annoying, they were in fact severe and humiliating. Segal never complained and yet he had become so sensitized that he would vomit at the sight of the syringe in anticipation of the side effects to follow.

We started an experimental immunotherapy program in hopes of inhibiting tumor growth. We were dubious about whether this would do much good, which meant that we had to reconsider surgery. Segal agreed to surgery more readily this time; months of nausea had convinced him that it might be less of an imposition on his freedom than chemotherapy had been. Also, in Segal's case there was a progression of the tumor. We asked the consultants in Houston to review his case.

July 9, 1973

The physicians in Houston recommended a surgeon at UCLA and Segal flew to Los Angeles to consult with him. They talked at length about the quality of life and the doctor told him that if the operation was a success, he might expect to have one and a half to two years of good life ahead of him. The doctor then showed him a graph based on the doubling growth rate of his tumor and assured him that without an operation he would be dead in 5.2 months. He also said that if they were unable to remove the total tumor, if the operation were a failure, Segal would not have long to live.

Although this doctor is a leading surgeon with extensive medical knowledge, he was playing prophet when he produced a figure like 5.2 months. Growth rates change; the nourishment to the tumor changes; and the body's immune system may affect these as well as other factors. Predictions have some validity, but no matter how much one knows about tumor growth rates, they provide incomplete data when the total situation of a patient is considered.

Segal didn't waver in his determination to die rather than become an invalid, so the operation became his only major option.

July 23, 1973

Segal and Janet came to my office to review all the points in favor of the operation before going to Los Angeles. Segal was satisfied that he and the surgeon had the same goals in mind, but I think Janet wanted to hear the arguments for herself. She was upset. I think she felt that her husband's case had not been properly handled and that he should have had the operation in January. Possibly his chances would have been better then. In any case, they now faced three possibilities. As Segal put it:

> I might die on the operating table, in which case everything is settled. They might make the resection and I'll get another two years, maybe more. Or they'll see that they can't resect and just close me up again. The last eventuality will be the hardest to live with, so I'm preparing myself for that. Besides, there's no choice now. I'm hurt and I'm tired. Without the surgery I'm going to be bedridden. Then I'll be dead.

July 30, 1973

The operation was performed and the tumor was not resectable. It appeared to be invading the liver and was highly friable. An attempted resection could have led to fragmentation, causing rapid spread of the malignancy.

My wife and I flew to Los Angeles the next day to be with Segal and Janet. When we entered the room, Segal was alert and cheerful, but when Janet and Isadora left his expression changed. He said, "Ernie, that was the last try. You begin to hope and that breaks you. All a man has at the end is his dignity."

We talked for a long time, and he told me about an experience he had had on a recent trip to Point Barrow, in Alaska.

> I've seen any number of pictures of the tundra and the Arctic wastes, but until I was up there I had not visualized how frightening, how truly frightening it is to be up there. The size is beyond conception. It isn't like the photographs, with borders. It's without borders. It's without words. I chartered a small plane and flew across the North Slope for hundreds of miles. There is nothing— no life, no polar bears, just snow. You can walk for eighteen hundred miles over the pole and down into Siberia. There is just nothing out there. I thought of the foolishness—or the incredible bravery—of the men in 1903 who started out across the ice cover, risking death. I've been close to death, but it's one thing to be there all of a sudden and not to whimper, and it's another to march across a plain resolutely, knowing that when you get there, you drop off. And its another yet to know that you are marching across the plain to the edge, but kind of blindfolded so that you get to see only occasionally. Treatment is that experience. It's marching across a plain resolutely, sometimes blindfolded, which is when you are receiving treatment or are in a remission or whatever; but

sometimes just seeing that you are getting closer. Suddenly the blindfold comes off and you are really close and it comes as a surprise. That is why people become freaked by their experience with treatment. And that's how people break. It's the uncertainty. There are lots of people who could march there with certainty and with dignity. But there will be a breakthrough on the horizon, which is now so close, and it will suddenly be extended—perhaps to infinity. How many times can people take that? I don't think I can take it, and I consider myself a very strong person.

Mid-August 1973

Segal had phenomenal recuperative powers. After the exploratory laparotomy (abdominal surgery), he was eating the following day and flew home three days later. That evening, five days after surgery, he attended a fund-raising party for the Friends of Cancer Immunology (FOCI) in San Francisco, brought several of his friends, and spent four hours helping to raise funds for cancer research. I am sure he was exhausted afterwards but that was his style—to maintain a high standard of performance.

I visited Segal at home late one afternoon. He had tried to keep up his active pace—a day each in New York, Washington, Denver, and New Orleans; but he was forced to take a day off because he was feeling so weak. He said,

> I'm becoming a kvetch, Ernie. But it's hard to do otherwise. I hope that Janet doesn't remember me as one. It's shocking to think that one has nine years of marriage, and a partnership, and that the last week is what people will remember you for. Of course I don't believe that, but I think the last week is an important week. I want Janet to remember me as I am today, not as I might be, should I become a weakly weeping kvetch. I don't want my children to remember me that way, either. I don't want to be that way. I demand it of myself. And I'll not let anyone deny it to me.
>
> I told you that when I went to Los Angeles I had prepared for the eventuality that the tumor would be inoperable. It was the only possibility I thought about because I knew it would be the most difficult to manage. If I'd gone down there hoping, I'd have been destroyed. Afterwards, I was upset but not devastated; and I was mostly upset because Janet was, and because I was going to have a lot of pain and discomfort for a couple of weeks when I might have been well. If you don't have much time, a couple of weeks is valuable.

Segal talked again about the treachery involved in hoping (which it is clear that he did, despite himself), and of how people do not have the resources to repeat very often the process of gaining, and then losing, hope. He also spoke of the horror that chemotherapy had been for him.

It's an indescribably awful experience. It's like going every morning and having an injection of stomach flu. You do it every morning, and you do it yourself. It isn't like, "If I'd only worn boots, I wouldn't have caught stomach flu." You're going out to be whipped every day. You think people get depressed or are cowards because they're not willing to take it. But, goddammit, it takes away from you. When I think of the things I've gone through, I'm appalled. I don't know where I found the resources. I've got to be satisfied that I can still live with quality. I think treatment risks doing a great disservice to people who want not to be bothered any more. But that isn't the same as folding up with no hope and going into a catatonic state, waiting to die. That's obviously one kind of reaction. But there are a whole bunch of people who just don't want to futz around any more. They want to do their thing and then they want to drop dead. But treatment does terrible things. I could talk about the injections and get sick—actually throw up thinking about them—even though I haven't had them lately. A cerebral person like me doesn't want to be tied to a bodily function that affects his mind. The point is that you really change, Ernie.

The results of Segal's treatment were only fair, since chemotherapy merely slowed down the growth of his tumor. But his side effects were out of proportion to the strength of the drug. Sometimes anxiety or the anticipation of bad results from a previous experience can increase toxicity; and although Segal appeared calm on all occasions, he was undoubtedly conditioned by his prior toxic experiences. Conversely, a patient who approaches therapy with a positive attitude often has less toxicity.

After the operation in Los Angeles I had been worried about Segal's becoming despondent and had recommended that he talk with a psychiatrist.

You think I'm depressed. You're wrong. I'm not depressed, let me assure you. I talked to my friends since you suggested I get psychiatric help. They don't think I've changed at all. And I don't think so. You're projecting. I am not voicing a more positive or negative view than I otherwise would. Except as things become more negative, you demand more positivism. You respond to negative impulses with greater positive adrenalin. I don't respond more or less to negative impulses. I persevere. And that's an important difference between us. You are far more genuine than I am, and I admire you for it, but I don't think either of us would trade places.

Nevertheless, Segal was always aware of what pain and time could do to him. He kept open the option of suicide at the appropriate moment. I asked him if he thought he could do it.

I spent a lot of time thinking about that. I don't doubt my ability to do it, but it's a continuous battle between you and me to decide whose will is going to prevail. I have to guard against hoping too much. You might talk me into one treatment after another until I lose perspective. I fear I'll be worn down through a process of attrition which will involve on the one hand my physical illness but the result of which will be that my perceptions and my rationality will be impaired or distracted. Then I'll become like everyone else after a while—hanging on. The most rational, the most powerful, the most independent among us are subject to being worn down, the only difference being that some of us act at this point while some of us wait too long.

I don't think you would consciously wait too long to let me go, but your threshold is different than mine. And you don't know what it's like. It's like what Negroes call the Black Experience. You can't know what it's like to be black unless you really are a black. And it's not even enough to be black. You have to be black in a special situation.

I tried to reassure him by saying, "I've promised you won't suffer and that I'm not going to keep you alive when there's no hope."

But we have different senses of hope. I'm not going for a 5 percent chance. Maybe you would. I want to be sure it's the decision I'd make.

I didn't doubt that Segal could kill himself, yet this rarely happens among cancer patients. A person's capacity to endure seems to grow as the need arises.

Mid-September 1973

After the operation in July, Segal refused all further treatment, although the tumor grew steadily. Most days he worked an average of sixteen hours, but one day in September he returned early from a business trip because of a new pain in his back and chest. His spirits were low. He said, "Dying slowly is like psyching yourself to be executed tomorrow morning at dawn and learning at dawn that it's going to be put off for another day, and that goes on day after day. And it breaks the spirit."

Nevertheless, he agreed to have angiograms in preparation for the possibility of introducing chemotherapy directly into the arterial system that feeds the tumor. He also agreed to radiation treatments that might relieve his pain by shrinking the tumor.

November 27, 1973

The angiograms showed that the tumor was pressing against Segal's liver but had not yet invaded it; they also revealed the growth of a second tumor behind his heart. We gave him radiation for the second tumor but another method of dealing with such a tumor would have been to insert a tube in the aorta, the major artery in the body, and to apply chemotherapy directly to the tumor. This would have meant carrying around a pump with a chemotherapy reservoir and making frequent visits to the hospital. Segal's philosophy and self-image did not include that kind of dependence on tubes, and he vetoed the idea.

Radiation provided sufficient pain relief to enable Segal to work, even though his treatment schedule was sometimes upset by business trips. However, I think that the best medicine is not always the best medical care. It is more important that a patient have freedom to live and work.

Segal had by this time survived almost 5 of the 5.2 months predicted by his Los Angeles surgeon.

January 5, 1974

I asked Segal how he felt about the reprieve he was receiving through the radiation treatments.

It doesn't seem like a reprieve to me. It just means I'll live a little longer. I wasn't looking for a reprieve. I was looking for energy and achievement. A reprieve doesn't provide that.

I wanted to leave behind me a kind of statement. I thought I had plenty of time, but more achievement will be denied me. One achieves and makes statements on different levels. One of the statements we obviously make is our children and how they grow up, the chain of immortality they represent. That will be denied me. And even if they remember me, it doesn't matter. I won't have had the impact on Rebecca and Josh that the next ten to fifteen years would have meant. They will not be my statement.

Another statement is made in our work and what we accomplish in the marketplace of ideas, money, business, or whatever. When I walk down Montgomery Street, I think, "Some of these people will accomplish things. I won't." I have every reason to believe I would have achieved more in my work, but I've run out of time.

A third statement, which I think I have achieved, is that indefinable quality of being a good person. There are a lot of people who love me because I am really a pretty decent and interesting guy. That is important to me, the achievement of love.

I've run out of time because I've run out of energy. I'm in a holding action. It takes everything I have just to keep moving. It's difficult to maintain one's grace. If this year were a repeat of last year, I don't believe I'd go through it. It's no longer cancer and me. Each new treatment has removed me from the privacy of my own dealings with cancer. To you and the other doctors I'm just a tool. It's a war of attrition with constantly more troops. It's not my war any more.

Although Segal said he was worn down psychologically, he still strove for excellence and precision in his work and was, I am told, a catalyst in fostering these qualities in his associates.

Mid-February 1974

After neurologic consultation for progressive back pain, Segal entered the hospital for a myelogram. The diagnosis was recurrent tumor invading the sciatic nerve, so radiotherapy was reinstituted and provided some relief from pain. But when the radiotherapy was only partly completed, he decided to go home and receive the treatments as an outpatient. He never would stay in a hospital a minute longer than necessary.

In addition to giving Segal radiotherapy for pain relief, we tried to teach him how to give himself pain shots, but he was not sufficiently interested to become proficient. Even when his pain was severe, he would sometimes postpone receiving a shot as a test of strength.

Late February 1974

When a person has cancer and life can no longer be measured in quantity, quality becomes the objective. Segal achieved this quality before he had cancer, but he continued throughout treatment to make the most of each day. During the last two weeks of February he became too weak to go to the office and spent most of his time in a rented hospital bed in a sunny corner of his living room. He enjoyed being at home with his family and would invite his friends over for cocktails, sometimes holding meetings or advising friends and colleagues.

He continued to go to the hospital for radiotherapy treatment, but as the pain increased, he became more of an invalid. Going to the bathroom, three rooms away, was a chore. He almost required pain medicine for the trip. The back pain increased; the muscle spasms became intense, wracking his entire body. I remember being called by Segal, who was almost in tears, at five o'clock one morning to come over and give him a shot. He received his evening shots from a psychiatrist neighbor, and with those, the pills, and the muscle relaxers, he made one day at a time.

Finally the trips to the hospital for radiotherapy became too difficult and treatment was discontinued.

Segal might possibly have gained some extra weeks or months of life from another round of chemotherapy, but he did not want any more treatments. He was tired. In one year he had had five months of intense chemotherapy, surgery, radiation therapy, and immunotherapy—the whole breadth of medical treatment for cancer. But he did say that the past year and a half had been worth it because he had the chance to enjoy his family and to watch the personality of his small son develop.

March 9, 1974

I stopped at Segal's home and found him sitting up in bed, bright-eyed, talking excitedly on the telephone. When he hung up, he looked around the room at Janet and me and appeared immensely pleased about something. He had recently revised the charter for a large Eastern city, and the call had been from the chairman of a Senate committee, informing him of legislative approval and congratulating him on the excellence of his work. (Segal had worked so hard and so well that few of his business associates ever knew he had cancer.)

Isadora and I decided to have a luncheon to celebrate Segal's success. The weather was unusually nice, and Janet and Segal invited several of their friends. We sat around eating and drinking wine, discussing the President's problems and other topics. It was one of those memorable days, and Segal was at his best.

But during the next three days Segal's debility increased. He would lapse into a partial coma and then reawaken to capture additional moments with Janet and his children, his mother, and his friends. He said he appreciated more and more during those weeks having those he loved constantly with him. And although he did not want help, he needed it and accepted it graciously.

March 13, 1974

Janet was with him, and his mother and children were near, when Segal lapsed into a coma and died, at home, on the morning of March 13.

He succeeded until the last several weeks in not allowing cancer to interfere with his way of life. Even then, while physically spent from pain and the sedation of pain-relieving drugs, he managed to finish two important projects. And he kept his sense of humor.

Segal also maintained his self-respect and autonomy in his relationship with me, refusing to suffer many of the humiliations and indignities of a person who would sell his soul for a few more pills or days of life. It is impossible for the self-image of a man like Segal not to suffer from dying slowly; but Segal did not break in the end, as he had feared. He met his challenge with courage and accomplished what he most wanted, to live and die with style and dignity.

6 · Joan Stansfield

I think perhaps self-awareness, self-concern, and self-love without egomania are things we should all be able to reach without first running into a brick wall. It shouldn't take a fatal diagnosis to make us look at things squarely and deal with them straight on, or stop lying to ourselves. But I'm afraid for most of us it does. I think I've straightened myself out in the areas where I was deluding myself. In fact, I discovered while I was in the hospital that I'm a stronger person than I might have anticipated. I am just a bit gutsier than I thought, and I'm delighted to know that.

Joan lived in San Francisco on a steep hill lined with vividly and variously colored Victorian houses, but the apartment she shared with her three children was somewhat small for their needs. Mornings were hectic, with Joan rushing to her job downtown. Mike, eighteen years old and a senior in high school, usually had an early morning class, so it fell to twenty-year-old Derek to take his sister, Cathy, who was five, to the day-care center on his way to classes at City College.

A frequent visitor at the apartment was Joan's ex-husband, Jack, who lived several streets away, while a ringing telephone often signaled a frantic call from Joan's mother, who lived alone across town. Joan would have been living with Jack if he had not had a drinking problem, and she might have lived with her mother if she had not been a smothering, overconcerned parent. As it was, Joan's emotional endurance was often severely tested as she sought to maintain an equilibrium in these relationships.

The consequence of her husband's problem was that Joan had worked for years to provide steady financial support for her children. At forty-two she still had all these responsibilities and, in addition, her daily routine was affected by cancer and cancer therapy. She worried about the future in terms of her responsibilities because she knew she would probably die of the disease.

Joan is the most reliable and eloquent witness to her own experience with cancer, and I hope her story, assembled from tape-recorded conversations, will give some idea of the kinds of difficulties a cancer patient with family burdens may encounter. But more than that, in Joan we see a person faced with terminal cancer who discovered untapped resources of strength and flexibility and who as a result refused to let cancer claim more than the necessary portion of her time and energy.

I waited quite a while before consulting a physician because four and a half years ago I had a similar irritation that forced me to stop nursing my daughter, Cathy. When the inflammation reappeared, it was much easier to assume it was a recurrence of that problem rather than something more serious. However, a time came when I knew. I knew because I had no pain, and I was aware that a malignant growth is often characterized by an absence of pain. I simply had a feeling of great sickness; and when I finally did have pain, my breast cancer had metastasized.

Since the diagnosis, the changes in my attitude have been subtle. I'm not even sure it's good for me to discuss them because I think one can analyze almost anything out of existence. But I remember that I wasn't particularly content with my life. I had problems with my mother and my ex-husband and I was certain that illness would be more than I could handle. When I realized I was going into the hospital, I wanted to give up altogether. Yet I'm a fairly cheerful person and, given a choice, I prefer to look on the better side of a situation. So after surgery, when I was able to assess my position, I decided, "All right, I have cancer. I will live with it. I won't necessarily die of it."

I think my father had something to do with that decision. We were very close, although I don't remember a great deal about him except that he loved gardening, hiking, and camping. When we went walking together on Sundays, he always made a walking stick for me. And my friends adored him because he was one of those fathers who would squat down to their level when he spoke to them.

He contracted Hodgkin's disease when I was five years old, and it must have been pretty advanced at the time of diagnosis because he collapsed and couldn't speak. I have always been in the habit of thinking that he died of cancer, but you know how little flash cards settle themselves down in the back of your brain? Well, last week I flashed on the thought that my father did not die of cancer. Although he had been given a year to live, he actually lived for seven years altogether after receiving radiation therapy. He died eventually of coronary thrombosis. So I suddenly thought, "My father did not die of cancer; I do not have to die of cancer. That's a point to concentrate on."

Another quite different influence in my past that has helped me was a certain fatalism acquired from my Scots Presbyterian upbringing. Although intellectually I now reject much of what I was taught, I still respond emotionally to the concept of God's will. What will be will be. I knew that when breast cancer metastasizes, it may go to the lungs, then to the rib cage or to the bone marrow, which is pretty bad and pretty ugly. Nevertheless, if you're going to have cancer, what a great time to have it! This is a real breakthrough period in cancer research, and if I don't make it until they find a cure, that's my problem.

I think I'm pretty good at not lying to myself. Maybe I'm too good at recognizing reality, but while I was in the hospital deciding to live with cancer, I learned about priorities. There are a great many concerns which have gone way down on my list. My mother, for one. She's a weeper and a sufferer; the violins are going all the time. After my operation she demanded of the doctor, "How long will it be?" He, thinking she meant how long would I be away from work, said "Six weeks." While I was coming out of the anesthesia, I could hear her on the telephone beside my bed informing everyone we knew that "Joan has six weeks to live."

In our relationship I am the mother and she is the child, although she rationalizes her dependence as "Joan needs me." It has been that way since my father died when I was twelve and she began acting out saving him by dragging me off to all kinds of clinics. About every six months I had to have a complete physical examination. She was sure there was something terribly wrong with me and that she would save me. I see this now; I wasn't aware of it at the time except that I knew I wasn't ill. But by the time I was sixteen, just graduating from high school, I think I must have been quite close to a breakdown just from being hassled by this widow who was going through her own changes, a sort of prolonged menopause. A very wise friend took me to her gynecologist and I was given a series of B_1 treatments which really helped me.

My mother is a hysteric personality and that kind of person usually creates a very inhibited child, which I was. What I needed was a sense of her confidence in me, but she could not give that; it's so easy to control people when you make them feel inept.

Now she is partly senile and lives in a past of forty years ago. When she first moved to San Francisco, I would go with her every Sunday to a nearby Congregational Church where the congregation is composed largely of retired people her own age. They made overtures of friendship, which she rejected because of her need to live her life through me. Now she is lonely but some people can be lonely anywhere. She feels left out, the self-sacrificing mother, the only one who can help, so the boys and I humor her and try to make her feel better. However, when I'm around her, I'm constantly reminded of how ill I am. She phones me every morning and says, "You poor thing." I am the cross she has to bear and she is helping me. Oh, is she helping me! With help like that, I don't even need cancer.

The other family problem which has descended in my list of priorities is my ex-husband's alcoholism. We separated for the second time six months after Cathy was born because I didn't want to go through that again with her. In the early years of our marriage I know I did all the wrong things, but then we both had therapy and I realized I was playing doormat and a lot of other roles, because alcoholism is a great game. Yet it is almost impossible not to become involved, to remain objective while someone stomps around and breaks up the furniture.

But we try to be objective, and the boys have a good feeling for Jack. They accept their father for what he is and for what he is able to give. He taught them both music; he worked with them in scouting; and even before that we were into camping, hiking, climbing, and all that. So they are able to be grateful, to recognize and enjoy the good qualities and just swing with him when he is unable to function.

Although I cannot live with Jack, I still have strong feelings of respect and admiration for his positive qualities, and I trust him more than anybody I know, which is why I was able to let him help me last year when I was in the hospital. He is fantastic in a crisis situation. He moved in with the children, gave financial aid, moral support, and all kinds of things. Day-to-day is his problem, accepting responsibility on a continuing basis. It's all such a colossal bore because alcoholics are so extremely predictable.

He now recognizes his drinking as something he must deal with; and although this is a problem that affects me deeply, it is one from which I must withdraw. I cannot help him.

With the change in priorities, it's me first, then Cathy, and then the boys, because they are old enough to be on their own. Yet I've learned more from them than from anyone else; I'm pleased to have known them and to be their mother.

Cathy was unplanned and this whole situation seems especially unfair to her. I feel I owe her a little bit more. But feeling sorry for her when she does not understand why we feel sorry for her is the most destructive thing I can think of. The boys know my cancer is terminal, but Cathy knows only as much as she can understand. She sees the television spots of the American Cancer Society on television and announces, "You have that too," as though it were a status symbol. She doesn't know it's fatal, but she knows it is something serious and that everyone is trying to find out about it.

Actually we don't talk very much about cancer; life goes on pretty normally, and the domestic chores get done. The boys get their own breakfasts and Derek takes Cathy to the day-care center, where I pick her up in the late afternoon. She and I go to the supermarket after that, although I often feel weak in my legs by then and have to lean on the shopping cart for support. We all help with cooking dinner and doing dishes, but extra projects such as covering the chair in the living room just don't get done. My principal problem is fatigue. I find it very frustrating that I doze off as I sit down to read in the evening.

Otherwise, cancer has not altered my life in any major way. I miss backpacking and other physical activity but I can live with that. I can also live with this nap of red fuzz on my head and this wig which doesn't resemble my own hair—and even the prosthetic device that gives me a bust line.

The only thing I find debilitating is dealing with people who make unfair emotional demands. Then I begin to get a physical reaction—sweat and a sense of weakness. I actually sweat and that's a nuisance with this wig, because it gets damp and then when I go outside it gets cold. I kind of resent that, but I hope it doesn't show because it's no one's fault; yet I think that is when I am aware of my illness, when someone makes a demand that I don't feel I can fulfill or that I choose not to fulfill. When the demand is really unreasonable, my reaction is that I don't have time for that kind of nonsense. Fardels I can bear, fools I won't.

I have always tried to live one day at a time, but I think I'm better at it now. My job is fairly stressful—a hassle, really. As supervisor of telephone representatives in the Customer Service Department of a major health plan, I build case loads for twenty employees and handle the inquiries and complaints they are unable to deal with. Although I enjoy the people I work with, and dealing with the public, the organization itself has been invaded by systems engineers and efficiency experts who do not understand the concept of service, in which quality should be valued over quantity. I try to handle all this well without going overboard, but I'm a thorough person and don't like to leave things hanging. So I try to conserve—not so much physical energy as coping and imaginative energy, my resources that are most affected by my disease and my therapy.

Chemotherapy began the day I left the hospital in 1972. My liver was enlarged and invaded by cancer and I had early signs of jaundice. That first drug reversed the entire process and I became normal, but after five months I reached toxicity. The side effects were severe. I was dropping things and having memory lapses, so I kept, at my oncologist's request, a record of my symptoms over a period of twelve days:

Wednesday,   March 15   Heavy gas pains, no stool. Took laxative.

Thursday,   March 16   Diarrhea. Stay home. Sleep.

Friday,	March 17	Work half day. Ill; no stool. Laxative.
Saturday,	March 18	Sleep until 2:00 P.M. Perk up in the evening.
Sunday,	March 19	Sleep most of the day.
Monday,	March 20	Stay home in bed.
Tuesday,	March 21	Pain, ill. Work half day.
Wednesday,	March 22	Heavy gas pains; no stool. Laxative.
Thursday,	March 23	Diarrhea all day. Stay home. Try to sleep.
Friday,	March 24	Work all day. Sleep from 7:30 P.M. Friday to 11:00 A.M. Saturday.
Saturday,	March 25	Grocery shop at very slow tempo. Drag through day. Perk up in evening.
Sunday,	March 26	Slept nearly all day. Washed out. Some diarrhea. Splitting headache.
Incidentals:		Mouth sores in corner, spreading inside. Slow healing of minor scrapes. Greatly lowered pain threshold. Memory failure. Heartburn. Gas.

At that point my therapy was changed to another drug. The first one had done its job; the second maintained my remission. Two weeks after the changeover, I felt alert, my memory improved, and I was much more cheerful. I had been constantly aware of illness on the first drug but now I thought of myself as a well person who gets tired easily or who has pain sometimes. Unless I run into the weepers, I forget I have cancer.

Speaking of weepers, yesterday a difficult customer was directed to me for special handling. He wanted reimbursement for a flight he had taken to Tijuana for Laetrile treatment, but such coverage was not included in his contract. I needed some information from him but he was too angry and self-pitying to cooperate. Finally he blurted out, "Listen, lady, I've got terminal cancer." So I replied, "Isn't that a coincidence! So have I." Needless to say, he began to cooperate and even invited me to join a group of cancer patients that meets regularly and issues a newspaper on the latest drugs. I can understand going that route, but I choose not to.

Today I had an appointment for chemotherapy review, so after lunch I took a bus to the office of my oncologist. Of my three doctors—internist, surgeon, and oncologist—he is the one on whom I am most dependent right now. It's interesting, though. Neither he nor either of the other two ever said, "Why didn't you come to us sooner?" They just analyzed the situation and did their best once I got there.

The first time I met my oncologist, Dr. Rosenbaum, I was still in the hospital. I liked him immediately. He was very matter-of-fact, very low key. I just liked him, liked his face. You can't explain reactions like that, but I'm quite sure that if I hadn't liked him, I wouldn't be responding in quite the same way to chemotherapy. And when I do have discomfort, I am better able to tolerate it because of the confidence I have in him.

I'm even pleased by the atmosphere in his waiting room. There is little chitchat among the patients, no gloomy comparisons of symptoms. This isn't the result of any directive from him. I think people behave the way they do because that's the way they are with him. It's a very subtle thing, as are all aspects of one's attitude toward living with cancer.

The first thing I do during an office visit is give my blood to Sophie, my personal vampire; then, since the wait may be a half hour or more, I lie on the examining table and take a nap.

The interval between office visits has varied from one to three weeks, but I'm a little uncomfortable with the three-week span. It isn't anything terribly inspiring that he says to me or that I ask him. It's just seeing him and "How are you?" and "You look great!" And he usually teases me about the wig. But I know he is frightfully busy and I always worry that I'm taking up too much time and asking too many questions. Therefore, I either write down the questions or get them firmly in mind so I can ask them quickly and absorb the answers, because those answers are terribly important to me.

When Dr. Rosenbaum was on vacation, I didn't get nervous, but I did cross streets very carefully. I didn't make any waves anywhere because I didn't have him to run to. Anybody could have helped, I suppose, but I felt a responsibility to behave myself.

I think if I had to define an effective physician, I would say one who sees and treats in each patient more than the physiological aspects of his problem. When Dr. Rosenbaum is planning a treatment program for me, I know he takes into consideration my various responsibilities and sources of tension and concern. For example, he changed my chemotherapy so I could continue working and keep my home together, and he has helped me arrange that my cousin become Cathy's legal guardian when I die.

We talked today about whether or not I should apply for Aid to the Totally Disabled.* Cancer that is neither cured nor controlled is considered ample qualification for receiving help, and I asked Dr. Rosenbaum whether he would consider it ethically feasible to recommend me. He said he wanted me to understand he was pleased with my progress but at the same time would be will-

---

* As of January 1974 a person can apply for Supplemental Security Income for the Aged, Blind, and Disabled. It is advisable, when possible, to apply for this aid and for Social Security Disability three to six months in advance of the need. A person who thinks he may qualify for such help, now or in the future, should ask his local Social Security office for further information.

ing to give the authorities the necessary medical information. The question is complex, however, and I'm not really good at making heavy decisions. I have a tendency to look at both sides very carefully and to conclude that either way will work. I guess I don't have a strong enough ego to say, "*That's* what I'm going to do." Although I have good disability coverage in my health plan, that would not go into effect until six months after I stop working. Social Security Disability benefits require a wait of five months. I have always worked to provide a steady, predictable income for my family and I have a responsibility to feed my children. Because of these financial considerations, I will have to weigh the pros and cons carefully. On the other hand, if I'm going to go on Disability eventually, why not do it now when I'm functioning fairly well? I'm good at self-starting and could accomplish a lot without the discipline of an 8:00 to 4:30 routine.

Yet I have never been a well enough organized person to have a life goal. I think living a useful life is more important to me and that again is why the decision about Disability is so important. Can I be more useful to Cathy and the boys if I go on Disability and am available, doing things I consider important, or is it better to go on in one's little rut? I think you can overdramatize this a bit. One simply needs to make a choice. I could walk out the door right now, get hit by a truck, and not have done all my great life-dream things.

I mentioned Disability to my mother, very casually, as a possibility only, because I didn't want her to freak out again and think I had only two weeks to live. Her immediate reaction was "Of course you won't be able to make it financially, so I'll move in," at which point I decided, "Forget Disability for the time being."

I don't know what course my illness will take. I have told Dr. Rosenbaum I have very strong feelings about the slow and dirty aspects of dying with cancer. Although I have no religious or other strong feelings about suicide, I am constrained by a non-suicide clause in my insurance policy. I definitely believe in euthanasia, yet if I were a physician I don't know whether I'd be capable of making a professional decision. I just know what my own personal emotional feelings are, and I can't bear the thought of putting my family through what I've seen so many families go through. It's all so pointless. It's all so stupid. It's an ego trip too. I don't want to be remembered as that stinking body lying on the bed for days and days, turning into a complaining, demanding thing. Because that's the kind of memory that sticks.

I remember when I was a child being taken to visit a maiden aunt who was sick. It was summertime in a small town in an old house, and she was dying in an upstairs room of cancer of the intestines. She only had a sheet over her because of the heat but the sheet was draped over a wooden frame so it wouldn't touch

the bones which were protruding through her skin. The weight of
the sheet would have been agony for her. I remember the stench
and I remember the revulsion. And I think of her when I think
of getting to the slow and dirty stage.

I have no fear, just an attitude about not rotting, and a desire
to protect my children from things that are unnecessarily unpleasant. But there is no point in thinking about that now. I'm not
there and can't predict what kind of strength I'll have for coping if
that time comes. I will have to do it day by day, as I do now.

"Now" is not so different from yesterday. I don't think I perceive color, sound, all the senses, more deeply, but I do relish
them more. Sunsets I have always enjoyed, but now I really wal-
low in a good sunset. But I don't think, "This may be my last sunset." I can't play that role. This may be an overreaction to my
mother and her "Sarah Bernhardt is alive and well" routine, but it
is also an attempt to be honest in my emotional reactions instead
of overdramatizing them. One is so Hollywood-oriented. People
with final diagnoses always do beautiful romantic things like going
off to Mexico. I am just aware that I take more time to enjoy
things, like walking on a raw day in San Francisco with a cold
wind in my face.

I have mentioned that one must often treat the family as well as the
patient. This was true of Joan's mother, for whom I could not help feeling sympathy. Elderly, arthritic, and nearly blind, she wanted to give
comfort to her only child. And she was fearful of her own lonely future.
During episodes when Joan was hospitalized, I felt her mother needed
comfort and compassion and I tried to reassure her of her usefulness
to Joan. At the same time Joan needed some respite from her mother's
constant attendance, some moments of peace in which to recover.

As with all my patients, Joan's life circumstances—the need to support her family and maintain a household—helped me to determine the
type of treatment she should receive. She could not continue to take a
drug that knocked her off her feet for several hours a day. She also
needed my steady interest and concern; and I think my availability and
our short, frank conversations provided this for her, as well as the
hope of achieving stability in her disease, which she did for many
months.

In a sense Joan required less emotional support from me than Mort
Segal. Where he needed encouragement to continue treatment, Joan
simply wanted advice and reassurance. Thus my role differs with each
patient, although it is not something I think about ahead of time. Patients tend to cast me in the roles they require, and I try to respond
appropriately as their needs become evident. Like them, I meet one
situation at a time, one day at a time.

7 · Louise Milner

"How could this happen to me?"

"It didn't happen to you, Mr. Milner. It happened to your wife," replied the surgeon. He had just performed a radical mastectomy on Louise Milner, aged twenty-eight. When Louise discovered the lump in her right breast a few weeks earlier, she had asked her husband how he would feel if she were to lose her breast. His quick reply stunned her: "I couldn't bear it. I can't stand cripples."

Today, five years later, Louise sits opposite me at my desk and moves carefully in her chair to find a comfortable position. Her right arm is swollen and half paralyzed from nerve damage. Skin metastases cover her chest, shoulders, and neck. Less than one lung is functional. She talks about her life before cancer and sighs, "I'll never get over losing my breast."

The eldest of three daughters of Russian immigrants, Louise was already a beauty in her teens. She received modeling offers, was envied and adored for her long blond hair, lovely face, and exquisite figure. She enjoyed a close family life but felt her parents were overprotective and wanted to be independent of them. Since "nice Russian girls" did not leave home and get their own apartments, marriage appeared to be the logical means of escape; and when Louise met David Milner, he seemed to have the proper credentials: tall, blond, a "Greek god," and an engineer. But after one year of marriage Louise, six months pregnant, fled to Los Angeles and got a divorce. David had spent most of his evenings gambling, often lying about where he had been, and he was hostile to the idea of having a child.

After her daughter, Sandra, was born, Louise began to model and dance professionally and to learn the techniques of staging fashion shows. During the next two years her career flourished and she was offered numerous jobs in the Nevada gambling resorts. It was while dancing in one of these clubs that she met, and married three months later, Gil Smithfield, a general practitioner from the area. Louise became his office manager, acting as receptionist, bookkeeper, and part-time nurse in addition to continuing her career of modeling and arranging fashion shows at the local clubs. She also ran a ballet school and a charm school. Life would have been ideal except that this time her husband's addiction was other women. Louise was distraught much of the time and a sense of inadequacy began to grow. "I even tried to model myself after each of his new lovers," she remarked. She tried to please at the same time that she felt she was being used; and she was therefore angry with herself and with Gil. A particularly notorious affair with a visiting celebrity precipitated a suicide attempt by Louise and resulted in plans for divorce.

Louise's first husband, David, read a vague account of these happenings in a gossip column, guessed that Louise was involved, and immediately wrote her to offer his support. They began corresponding. David expressed regret for his past behavior, spoke of his longing to be with his daughter, and reminisced tenderly about his love for Louise. Louise says she cared too much for Gil to feel she could stay away from him if she were alone. She needed someone—so, hurt and lonely, she divorced Gil and remarried David. The marriage seemed to be working until Louise discovered the lump in her breast.

It is not unusual to hear a beautiful woman complain that she sometimes does not feel loved for her true self. This was how Louise felt when David became impotent after her mastectomy. A day came when he moved out of the house, telling her he couldn't make love to "someone like that." David's view of Louise became her view of herself. She felt that she made people uncomfortable, that she was flawed, no longer desirable, and there followed a series of experiences which confirmed these facts for her.

Actually it had begun in the hospital. Doctors and nurses would glance into Louise's room and then hurry away, avoiding eye contact. She would call out to them, "Please come in. It's all right." But they quickly made excuses to leave.

One evening a resident, having perceived Louise's ostracism, went to her room and, with the best of intentions, told her she might cry if she wished. Louise informed him she was not ready to cry, but he urged her again. He was compassionate, but his analysis of Louise's emotional state was inaccurate; and he appeared confused when she failed to react according to his preconception of her.

Out of the hospital Louise observed the same tentative behavior in many friends and relatives. One friend would not visit her after the mastectomy for fear she would "catch" cancer. There were, of course, positive experiences too, kindness and concern from unexpected quarters. Nevertheless, Louise was generally demoralized and forlorn when she entered her surgeon's waiting room for a follow-up visit. In the waiting room was one other patient, a woman with only half a face. Louise became terrified, thinking, "My God! Am I going to die looking like that?" and burst into tears as she entered the surgeon's inner office. When she explained why she was upset, he berated her, "You baby! You don't have that kind of cancer." Louise did not know what kind of cancer she had, only that she needed reassurance. Then the surgeon told her to raise her arm as high as she could, and when Louise failed to raise it higher than her shoulder, he again became impatient. "It's got to be higher!" Louise said she was trying; he told her she was not. She wept some more and promised herself that by the next visit she would raise her arm high enough to strangle him.

When, by the next appointment, Louise was able to raise her arm and told him how angry he had made her, he crowed, "But you see? It worked! Your arm is up where it should be." Louise was not impressed. She felt he could have achieved the same result with a gentler approach.

Several weeks later Louise sat in another waiting room at a local hospital, where she had gone for a cobalt treatment. She passed the time chatting with a patient who, on hearing the purpose of Louise's visit, related lurid tales of the effect cobalt had on her girl friend's father's best friend. The friend had lost sixty pounds; his hair had fallen out; and he had had frequent blood transfusions. Louise was horrified at the time, but fortunately she found that she gained fifteen pounds, kept her hair, and needed no transfusions. She is now very definite about the adverse effect such tales may have on an inexperienced patient: "If I met someone who was going to have chemotherapy, I would not mention the possibility of nausea because that might produce a worse reaction than he might otherwise experience."

Louise also feels strongly that medical technicians ought to be allowed to discuss the results of tests with patients. There is usually a lapse of hours or days before a patient learns the results of the latest test from his doctor. It would be better, Louise thinks, to hear a white lie, a word of encouragement from the technicians, to reduce worry in that interval. "Worry is what makes you unable to sleep or eat, and much of the time it's responsible for depression. People are more frightened by the silence of those technicians than they would be if they'd just say everything is fine. No wonder people give up."

After her second divorce from David, Louise moved, with Sandra, into her parents' home in San Francisco. Her parents did everything they could to make Louise feel comfortable and welcome, but what she really wanted was a man to tell her she was still a desirable woman. Although the operation had revealed that her cancer had metastasized, Louise was in relatively good health, and she wanted to enjoy life. Again, however, the reactions of others did nothing to restore her confidence. She recalls an evening when her mother happened to be in her room while she was undressing. Louise had removed the prosthesis which fitted into her bra and replaced her breast, and her mother said, "Turn around, honey, so I can see your incision." But when Louise turned around, her mother gasped, "Oh, my poor baby," and burst into tears.

Nevertheless, during a visit to Los Angeles Louise summoned the courage to telephone a man she had dated between her marriages to David and Gil, a man who had kept in touch with her through the years and always assured her of unflagging devotion. They had lunch several times but Louise did not tell him about her operation or her cancer. Then one evening on his sailboat, as he was telling her of his affection and of his admiration for her beauty, Louise interrupted him. "Before you go any further, I want you to know that I have cancer and that I've had a breast removed." Louise reports that he catapulted to the other side of the boat, hitting his head on the boom, and stared at her. She told him to take her home, and she never heard from him again.

Back in San Francisco, Louise accepted invitations from time to time from men she found attractive. She was fearful of repeating the experience of Los Angeles, yet in different ways she did repeat it, over and over. She would go out with someone once or twice and then defensively blurt out her news. Protestations would follow that this "made no difference," but that was usually the end of the relationship. Louise now acknowledges that although she occasionally met with insensitivity, she was also insensitive in her bluntness, and she courted rejection in order to avoid future emotional pain. Her increased vulnerability only sharpened her defenses and reinforced her self-rejection and her loneliness.

Then Louise met Alex. His wife had died of cancer, and he was familiar with the disease. The word did not paralyze him. Louise says, "He was kind and serious, and we were compatible, a good couple. And I was very happy."

Two years passed in this way, until Louise suffered a recurrence of her disease. She spent a month in the hospital recovering from an oophorectomy and exploratory surgery, and during all that time she did not hear from Alex. Finally she phoned him. He announced he was getting married to someone else; he loved her, would always remember her, but he could not go through with her what he had gone through with his wife. Louise said later, "He really hadn't minded about the mastectomy; he was afraid of the cancer that was still in my body."

Louise did not date again. "It hurt my feelings too much. I couldn't take another rejection." She withdrew into the safer world of family and friends. But even at home there were problems. Her family was loving and devoted, but Louise felt they too were angry with her for being ill. She would try to allot the same time and energy to their activities that she had before, but when she became exhausted trying to please them, she was full of resentment.

During this time, the fourth year after Louise's mastectomy, cancer spread to her liver and lungs. Chemotherapy was begun and her initial response was good, with excellent control of the cancer; but after several months she was often nauseated and suffered from attacks of anxiety that developed into long periods of depression. She felt that she was a burden to her family and a bad mother to Sandra. "Do you have any idea how useless I am and how painful it is for me to live?" she asked several times. I tried to make Louise understand how important she was to Sandra and that the grandparents could never take her place, but her mood did not improve. Then I reduced and altered the chemotherapy, and although her mental anguish decreased, the disease itself began to progress slowly. Suddenly, in a moment of desperation, Louise cast her hopes in another direction.

Telling me she was going to Hawaii for a vacation, Louise flew to Tijuana for Laetrile treatment, even though she was familiar with the controversy over Laetrile's therapeutic value. Mort Segal spoke of the loss of hope that erodes the spirit; for Louise, too, the apparent failure of chemotherapy to stem the growth of her cancer destroyed her faith in conventional medicine.

In Tijuana Louise stayed in a hotel that offers a special menu for cancer patients who have come for Laetrile treatments. At the clinic itself, she recalls, there were six doctors, plus nurses and other staff; but in the waiting room there were never fewer than seventy-five people. For two months Louise visited this clinic and received Laetrile orally and by injection, but the doctors made no attempt to monitor her physical response. Specifically, no X rays were taken of her chest; and her disease continued to progress.

Although Louise experienced no improvement, she struggled to maintain a semblance of enthusiasm as an encouragement to the patients who had become her friends. They came to her when their own spirits were low, and Louise sadly recalls, "All those people around me were dying."

By the time Louise decided to return to San Francisco, she was critically ill. Almost the moment she came into my office she blurted out the truth about her absence. She was embarrassed and hoped she hadn't offended me by seeking other help, but I could understand what motivated her and I don't believe in worrying about the past. I put Louise in the hospital, where an X ray revealed that her right lung had collapsed into a cancerous mass and her chest cavity was filled with fluid. I then summoned a thoracic surgeon, who placed a drainage tube in her chest and removed five quarts of liquid. The right lung had atrophied and would never function again; the left lung was being invaded by cancer. She had progressive disease on her skin all across her chest, and more liver involvement. If an X ray had been taken of her chest while she was in Tijuana, it might have been possible to save part of her right lung.

I immediately began a new course of intense chemotherapy. Louise's hair did fall out this time and she again had side effects, but the rapid progression of the cancer was halted.

The experience in Tijuana had made Louise fearful of dying. She felt constantly short of breath and did not feel secure unless she was close to an oxygen tank. Several times she was hospitalized because she couldn't breathe, but these episodes were in reality anxiety attacks. One day she confided in me, "I think I'm going to die." I replied, "I don't think so. Why do you?" Then, to reassure her that I would always relieve her pain, I promised her, "I won't let you suffer." The reversals in her health and the length of her illness had predisposed Louise to misinterpretations; she thought my statement meant that she was indeed about to die, and she went home and spoke to no one for several days. Fortunately, the misunderstanding was cleared up in a subsequent telephone conversation, and Louise's spirits improved.

By and large, however, the months following Louise's return from Mexico were the most psychologically debilitating since her mastectomy. The progression of her malignancy had caused her to lose hope, and she again contemplated suicide. I could only hope that her fear of death and the strong prohibition against suicide in her Russian Orthodox background would deter her from resorting to such a measure. But a patient's state of mind is often his most destructive symptom, and I was therefore afraid that Louise might die soon anyway if her mood did not change. The effect that a patient's emotions have on his physical status is one reason why statistics cannot be relied upon. They simply cannot predict how a given individual will respond to a particular treatment for a particular type of cancer.

I explained to Louise that she had been taking a drug which might have caused some of her depression and anxiety and that we would stop using it. I also gave her an antidepressant. We talked again about how much Sandra needed her and how, if Louise could live well with cancer, this could be a legacy for Sandra. The downward trend of Louise's spirits was finally reversed—largely, I think, because I acted contrary to my medical preference by withdrawing chemotherapy and using hormonal therapy instead. This ran the risk of more rapid physical deterioration, but freedom from the drug's side effects gave Louise energy to meet her emotional needs. She said one day, "You don't know how much your telling me to 'cheer up, don't give up' is like food to me. When you tell me I have a future, I know you're not just saying it to pacify me. And that, to me, is more than anyone could do. It cheers me up for weeks."

Since her mastectomy, Louise had avoided most of her former associates in the fashion and design world. She did not want them to see her in her present condition, and she felt she had nothing to offer them any more. "I had to do something else," she recalls. And she did. With her right hand almost nonfunctional, she trained herself to work with her left. At first she could neither thread a needle nor write. Hemming a dress took hours. But gradually she became proficient and began to take pleasure in sewing and other crafts. She designed dresses and bathing suits with high necks and loose flowing sleeves for women who had had mastectomies. She made sand candles and macramé chokers, earrings, and nets for hanging plants. She painted in oils and began an organic vegetable garden in the backyard. With her creative energy thus channeled, Louise began to feel useful; she was delighted when her efforts gave enjoyment to others. At the same time she began to find more pleasure in reading and to study psychic phenomena and reincarnation. She does Alpha mind control and healing meditation every morning and evening and says that Alpha has changed her way of thinking about herself. "I used to demand perfection of myself and my friends. Now I am easier about everything. I also suddenly realized I didn't care what people thought of me, that I was a pretty nice person and shouldn't have been so hard on myself. Before, I always felt I wasn't doing enough. Now I know I did more than the average, and I've found I like myself. In Alpha you simply program yourself for positive thinking and action."

Thus by the spring of 1973 Louise's condition had stabilized and she was relatively content. Sometimes during her office visits she would share with me her complaints about her family and tell me their criticisms of her. I would remind her that when a person is ill over a long period of time, ordinary aggravations can be magnified to proportions that stun both patient and family.

Louise's experience seemed to parallel Ellen's to the extent that many people either ignored her illness or were oversolicitous. This was illustrated during and after a family vacation at their summer cabin.

Louise said, "They seemed to forget I was sick and would urge me to go to the beach one minute and take a hike the next. I would explain that I couldn't be in the sun for very long and they would offer to bring an umbrella. If I refused, they would say I was no fun any more, so of course I did all the things they wanted." Within two weeks she was rushed back to San Francisco by ambulance, barely able to breathe. It would be difficult as well as futile to assign blame. Louise knew she should not overexercise. At the same time it is easy to imagine a collective will on the part of sisters, nieces, and nephews to relive the carefree years and try to forget Louise's cancer.

In the hospital Louise was given sedatives, oxygen, and narcotics for her pain, and she slowly recovered. However, her self-pity at having cancer and a relapse, and her anger at herself for not being able to say "no," was projected onto her family and friends. I felt that since she had such anger, it should be vented, and I urged her to telephone the people with whom she was most angry and to explain her feelings and the reasons for them. Louise did this, and it helped. Speaking out about her feelings has become one of the means with which she now deals with cancer. Her family, finding it hard to take at times, calls her the "Queen Bee," and Louise readily admits that she is sometimes demanding, quarrelsome, and impatient. But this is at least an honest reaction, and an open one. She is not harboring any emotionally exhausting secret animosities.

At the same time that Louise was accusing people of indifference and insensitivity, she was furious with her mother for being overprotective and solicitous. "The first night I was in the hospital after that vacation, my mother came over with chicken soup and enough apples, bananas, and peaches to fill the drawer beside my bed. She made me call the commissary and order ice cream, cookies, and milk and wouldn't leave until they were delivered. The next night, when my IV tube was hurting, I pulled it out and she screamed at me. The house doctor came and said the tube had pulled clear of the vein, that the fluid was making my tissues swell and I had been right to pull it out. Then all day long, just as I was dozing off, she would telephone me. She phoned me eight times in one morning."

It is not difficult to understand a frantic mother who equates every drop of IV and mouthful of food with an improvement in health. I suggested to Louise that she gently ask her mother not to telephone so frequently, but Louise insisted this would hurt her mother's feelings. I therefore spoke to her father, who explained that Louise's mother was always hoping for a miracle and that fussing over Louise was just her way of trying to make one happen. I told him there were no miracles, that Louise needed good care and rest. After that Louise's mother retreated to some extent, and I hoped she understood that my meddling was done in the interest of her daughter's health. Even if Louise had been exaggerating, I felt that my first responsibility was to meet her needs and to let her know I would support her.

Besides her mother's calls, in her first two days in the hospital Louise received twenty-five calls from relatives and friends asking, "How are you?" Barely able to breathe, operating at 40 percent of normal lung capacity, Louise labored to reply to such questions. "People should ask something you can answer 'yes' or 'no' to, or they should just offer their sympathy and ask if there's anything they can do. What if I replied that I was getting blood transfusions, and that I was nauseated and in pain with a 105 fever?" The phone calls were irritating, but they provided reassurance that people cared, and they also became a means through which she could vent anger at her disease. She did not have the phone turned off.

Talking over these episodes with Louise reminded me of the day she came into my office and I asked her how she was feeling. She smiled and said, "Marvelous," and we continued with the examination. That evening I told Isadora, who had also talked with Louise that day, how pleased I was that she felt so well and was in such good spirits. My wife shook her head and replied, "Louise just said that to make you feel good. She told me she deliberately dressed up and made herself look good so you'd be pleased."

I needed to be reminded how much we doctors encourage deceptions like Louise's, in and out of hospital. Too often a patient feels he must tell his doctors, family, and friends what they want to hear. Gaiety and good sportsmanship are rewarded; complaining or frankness is shunned. It should be possible to say, "Thanks, I feel lousy," without having people disapprove or turn away.

Louise has managed her life very wisely since the family vacation and its aftermath. Naturally, her condition and her moods vacillate, but she has learned what to expect from herself and others; she has learned, as Ellen hoped cancer patients would learn, that she can have a lot to do with her own and other people's attitudes toward her cancer.

For instance, Louise was aware that, despite all the open grieving by her parents and relatives, Sandra had not cried for months and that she was having one bad cold after another. Louise took Sandra aside and told her that any time she wanted to cry it would be all right, that as long as Louise knew she was not physically ill, she would ask no questions. Sandra looked surprised, closed the door to her room, and cried for two days. She stopped getting colds and began to bring friends home from school for the first time in a year.

At first Louise was worried that her appearance might frighten or embarrass Sandra's teen-age girl friends, but instead she found them relaxed, refreshingly open, and easy to talk to. Louise showed them her wigless head and told them to call her "chrome dome." On successive visits, they measured the growth of her hair. They asked her what it was like to be dying and whether she was afraid, and they expressed their fears for themselves and their parents. At other times they simply shared their everyday problems about school and boy friends. Their candor delighted Louise, and she came to consider these relationships among her most valuable.

Sandra, who has just turned fifteen, spends hours asking Louise about Louise's own childhood. Louise has observed the traditional jealousy between some of her friends and their teen-age daughters, and she feels this has been circumvented in her relationship with Sandra, partly because of her cancer.

In December 1973 Louise went to a Christmas party at the company where she had been a designer and a model. She had not visited her former co-workers for five years, and they were thrilled when she accepted their invitation. The owner of the firm gave her a long, two-piece, royal-blue outfit with a matching fur collar and hat, which she wore to my office just before the New Year. Her hair had grown back. She was stunning. No one would have guessed she had cancer. Before rushing off to a New Year's Eve party, she let me take her picture.

Since that time, Louise has created a way of life around the often terrible limitations imposed by her disease. She is still on hormonal therapy, and her fears about pain have been mitigated by access to pain-relieving shots which I taught her to administer to herself. "I know the pain will go away when I want it to. And it's funny how that cuts the pain down. If you have to worry about how to control pain, it seems aggravated. But, more than that, I know you won't let me suffer with half my face gone. I was always afraid of being a vegetable, of being doped up and not knowing for months what was going on. I don't know how you'll do it, but I know you won't let that happen. And that gives me security."

Louise, sitting across from me at my desk, has brought several of her latest paintings to show me. She is pleased that I like them and remarks, "I remember your saying, 'Louise, you must fill each day and live each day.' I never really knew what you meant because as each day came along I would think, 'Tomorrow I'm going to do this, and next week I'm going to do that.' I was always planning what I was going to do tomorrow but never doing anything today. Now I fill every day so full, unless it's a day when I'm not feeling well, that I sometimes don't get to all my projects. Do you realize it's been five years since I began receiving medical treatment? And next week I'm going to Hawaii for a vacation." Louise smiles and adds, "I'm really going to Hawaii this time."

8 · John Peterson

John Peterson was referred to me in the spring of 1971, a year after undergoing surgery and radiotherapy for melanoma. An alert, youthful-looking man of fifty, he began in a direct manner to describe his experience with cancer. I sensed a feeling of sadness and discouragement, and as his tale unfolded, I understood why.

On his return from a vacation with his family in the summer of 1969, John noticed a lump on the side of his neck. It was hard, and approximately half the size of a Ping-Pong ball. It did not hurt, but it was unusual; and he could not avoid being aware of it as he shaved each morning. Although anything relating to doctors and medicine had always triggered strong anxiety in John, he did in this case consult his family doctor, who assured him the strange lump was a common occurrence, a cyst. He declined to treat it, saying it would go away of its own accord, and asked John to return in a couple of weeks for routine observation. John returned in two weeks, and a month after that, but always received the same advice.

The cyst failed to disappear as predicted, and John naturally began to wonder whether the diagnosis had been accurate. Since the doctor was also his friend and had consistently reassured him, John was reluctant to bother him again. But when his friend became ill for a short time the following January, John took the opportunity to consult another doctor in the same office. This doctor was equally certain the lump was a cyst but suggested they go ahead and check it out by removing it surgically. He then referred John to a surgeon at the local hospital. After meticulously probing the spot, the surgeon announced, "Yes, we might as well remove it. These cysts can get nasty."

John did not look forward to the prospect of being unconscious and letting another person cut into his body. Moreover, he remembered a minor operation he had undergone as a small boy. The anesthetic wore off before the operation was finished, leaving John frightened and distrustful. However, he was now an adult, and he was pleased with the approach of the two doctors. Accordingly, he arranged to take a day or two of vacation from his job as assistant manager of a nearby lumber yard. The time would be well spent if the troublesome cyst could be removed. He entered the hospital on a Tuesday afternoon in January 1970 to prepare for minor surgery the following morning.

It was almost dark outside the hospital window when John awoke from the anesthetic on Wednesday afternoon. He tried to turn his head to survey his surroundings, but movement was painful and difficult. He touched his neck where the cyst had been. The bandaging seemed excessive, and the soreness surprised him, but he assumed this to be routine. Nevertheless, as a precaution he groped for the call button and told the nurse on duty he would like to talk with the surgeon as soon as it was convenient, half apologizing that he merely wanted reassurance that everything was all right.

A dinner tray was placed before John. He found it difficult to bend his head downward and consequently had to lift his plate to eye level to see what was on it. He picked at his food until his wife, Sue, arrived. She too was surprised at the degree of soreness and apparent extensiveness of the operation. At John's request she asked the nurses whether the surgeon would be coming by that evening. They told her they had left a message with his answering service and would probably hear from him shortly, although Sue guessed they were having trouble locating him. In any event, Sue and John were confident that he would appear before John's release on Thursday morning.

But the following morning the surgeon neither appeared nor telephoned instructions for John's dismissal from the hospital. As a result, each time a footstep or a voice echoed in the corridor, John glanced expectantly toward the door. His uneasiness grew as he repeated to himself the comforting litany, "It was just a cyst. Nothing could have gone wrong. The surgeon's a very busy man."

The nurse who brought John's breakfast and medication assured him that the tenderness in his neck was normal, but when he asked where the surgeon was or whether the operation had gone well, she suddenly appeared ignorant of his case. John's anxiety sharpened. As each hour passed, it became increasingly difficult to convince himself he was a victim of oversight or neglect. He could see that the nurses were sympathetic as well as nervously evasive; and when Sue joined him for dinner that evening, she also appeared anxious.

By dawn on Friday John realized he dreaded the surgeon's visit. The day before, passing footsteps had made him start in hope. Now he was relieved when they continued down the corridor. He lay still and waited.

He must have dozed off. A doctor he did not recognize was standing beside his bed. "Mr. Peterson, I'm the surgeon who assisted at your operation. Your surgeon had to leave town for several days and therefore asked me to speak to you. I'm going to be very frank with you, Mr. Peterson. You have incurable cancer. It's melanoma."

John had never heard of melanoma, and said so, whereupon the assistant surgeon told him, "A biopsy of the cyst reveals that you have a vicious type of malignancy, one with a highly unpredictable growth pattern. We're planning a more extensive operation next week, but I must warn you that just when you think you've got it all, it pops up in another area." Sometime during this recitation, John realized that his surgeon must have suspected he had cancer and failed to warn him. He began to cry, but the effort caused pain around his incision. Hesitantly he asked the doctor to tell Sue the diagnosis so she would receive a clear explanation of his disease and his prospects.

The second phase of the operation was performed a week after John was told he had melanoma. This surgery was more radical than the first and involved the removal of surrounding muscles.

John remained in the hospital another ten days and rested at home for a week before returning to work, his neck still in bandages. His family and friends were astonished at how quickly he got back on his feet. Radiation treatment was planned as a preventive measure to destroy any cancer cells the surgery might have missed, but such treatment cannot be given until a surgical wound has healed. In spite of his determined recovery, John's incision was particularly slow in healing, so it wasn't until six weeks after the second surgery that he began weekly trips for treatment to a radiotherapist in San Francisco. The therapy lasted three months, and on the days he made the two-hour round trip he still managed to work at least half a day.

On the importance of work in his life John once told me, "Work is all I know. I grew up during the Depression and my family was poor. I've worked since I was old enough to pull a grocery cart. I worked during vacations, after school, and on weekends. I even worked during the gym period at school. Consequently I never learned to play and never participated in sports like other children. Now, all these years later, I'm not content if I'm not working."

But John had other pleasures besides work. They may even have been accentuated by his cancer experience and the unpredictability of a recurrence. Sue is certain that the possibility of his melanoma's returning was always at the back of his mind, but she remembers that he was cheerful and tried hard to live each day. Looking back at this period of their lives, she recalls that they made more trips and in some ways enjoyed themselves more than in the years before cancer disrupted their lives. This was also partly due to their circumstances, the increased freedom of having their two older children on their own and the two younger ones almost ready for college. They spent much of their time improving their home inside and out, painting, rebuilding, and gardening. "We're both orderly people. We like things to be nice," John explained. The few hours when they weren't working at their jobs or on their home, they listened to their stereo, with the added pleasure of knowing their older son was studying to be a concert pianist.

In December 1970 Sue and John observed their thirtieth wedding anniversary and planned to celebrate by taking a long-hoped-for trip to Italy in the spring. Regrettably, the worst occurred in February 1971, when a new lump appeared near the site of the original tumor, only a year after the diagnosis of melanoma. Sue canceled their reservations and John re-entered the hospital for tests.

The surgeon who had performed the first operation had moved to another city, but the former assistant surgeon was available. He performed a biopsy and removed the tumor. He then told John he might have to lose his right arm, although later he changed his mind, saying that since the cancer had probably spread to other areas, removal of his arm would only cause extra pain and discomfort. "If I were you," he said, "I'd go home and forget about treatment. Your cancer has spread too far. Chemotherapy will only make you miserable during your remaining life. I've seen cases like this before."

John did go home, but he needed to take action against the surgeon's harsh pronouncement. That need brought John back to San Francisco to consult his radiotherapist, who referred him to me.

From the day of our first meeting and our talk about his background, his present life and work, and his discouraging encounters with two physicians, I knew my first goal must be to try to inspire hope. Thus I talked about control of his disease, about the possibility that the growth of his tumor might be slowed down or arrested. I told him how chemotherapy and experimental immunotherapy had led to improvement in many cases of melanoma; but I could not, of course, make any promises of cure. "I can only tell you what realistic results we can hope for. You can't quit until you've tried," I urged. John nodded, but because of all he had been told, faith in treatment would come only with success. For the moment his sadness prevailed over all my reasoning.

John consented to a program of experimental immunotherapy in the spring of 1971. He subsequently experienced periodic brief episodes. of high fever, flu-like symptoms, and a rash as a consequence of BCG immunotherapy, but the tumors in his neck were significantly reduced in size. Several months later frequent nausea took away his appetite; he tired easily and lost weight. Yet despite these discomforts tumor growth was controlled for over a year. John's desire to fight was sustained because he was able to work full time. This was evidence that he was not going to deteriorate as rapidly as had been predicted, evidence that in turn reinforced his courage to continue.

In the summer of 1972 John, Sue, and their two younger children made a trip to Canada. Just after their return, we discovered John's tumors had begun to grow again. Concurrently he began to dread the side effects of the drugs; and as his anxiety increased, he began to have attacks of nausea before treatment. In addition, he had pain in his right shoulder and numbness in his fingertips.

A month later, in September 1972, we discovered that John's disease had progressed to his lungs and liver. This meant that immunotherapy had ceased to forestall tumor progression, so we initiated a program that combined immunotherapy with chemotherapy. Unfortunately, the addition of the chemotherapy produced a stronger reaction of nausea than before, with the result that, in anticipation of his injections, John often vomited before reaching my office. But the chemotherapy also achieved a remission for several months.

Treatments were scheduled at two- to three-week intervals, and the accompanying nausea, which always humiliated John, lasted two days. A greater humiliation was experienced the following spring when his cancer once again advanced and the side effects from a new chemotherapeutic program forced him to cut his work day from eight to five hours. The forces of physical decline, side effects from treatment, and severe depression and anxiety merged and began to shatter his self-image.

John now left the office at three o'clock each afternoon. Tired rather than sleepy, he lay on his bed, often too weak to get up yet too nervous for sleep, trying to remember ever having been in bed at four o'clock in the afternoon. He felt defeated and ashamed. Angry with himself, he was easily annoyed with others. Unhappy at being, as he saw it, a burden rather than a sustaining force, he became less communicative. The days were long and monotonous.

One day during an office visit Sue, John, and I talked about the additional time John now spent at home, and I asked him if he had any hobbies or interests.

He replied, "All I've ever done is sleep, eat, and work. I have no hobbies. I don't read. Television bores me. I don't play cards. I do enjoy listening to the stereo, but you can't do that all the time. I want to work in the garden or go back-packing with my younger son, but I'm no longer able to do those things. And I see all kinds of things to do around the house, such as washing the windows, but I have no strength for that either. Consequently I'm depressed and everyone irritates me —Sue, the children. I no longer have any patience."

"How do your children react to your illness?" I ventured.

"I think they take it as a matter of course. Sometimes I even wonder if they're concerned about it. They don't help at home. They don't even clean up their rooms. The children of today are wrapped up in themselves. They've been spoiled.

"I wanted our children to have the education I didn't have," John continued. "I held down three jobs at one point. I worked at night so they could have all the extras, but the result is that they've never learned to do things. They aren't lazy—they're hard workers—but they've never known want. They've never known what it was to give every extra penny they earned for the support of the household."

Here Sue intervened. "It's difficult for John to put himself in the children's place, to understand that they see the world from a different perspective than he does. They're good children, but times have changed.

"John's mother became very ill when we were first married. As a matter of course John spent his summer vacation with her and took care of her while she was down and out."

"In this day and age it just isn't there," John sighed.

I met the Peterson children a few weeks later. We discussed the progression of their father's cancer, and his prognosis. They said they would do anything to relieve his anxiety and lessen his pain, that they felt helpless in the face of medical failure and advancing disease. Coupled with their frustration was the emotional fatigue of witnessing suffering that changes little from day to day. When disease is acute, or illness sudden, medical change in a patient may be rapid and dramatic. With a chronic illness such as John's, a patient's suffering may begin to be taken for granted by those around him.

John's children needed the distraction of school, friends, and sports. They also understood their father's need for encouragement and sympathy. I have often witnessed this particular conflict of needs, the solution to which lies in mutual understanding. To deal with impending loss, those close to a patient need to pursue their everyday activities, to establish and maintain an ongoing life. At the same time the help they give their loved one can be mutually rewarding. The patient receives emotional support while the family members fulfill their need to show their love.

During the late spring and early summer of 1973, John was given several combinations of chemotherapy, with little success. Each failure to achieve another remission led to a further decrease in physical stamina and deeper depression. His shame at not doing his share of the work consumed him, and as a consequence he withdrew even more into himself.

One day he said, "I used to help Sue, but now I come home at night and I'm unable to do anything."

"He used to do a lot," Sue confirmed.

"Since the kids don't always pitch in, Sue's stuck fixing dinner, getting it on the table, and doing the dishes. Then she has to correct papers for her second-grade class, which means she doesn't get to bed until after midnight."

I wondered whether it would be possible for them to spend more time together, but Sue responded, "We spend lots of time together, but we could spend better time. John is lonely, and I'm lonely. And we shouldn't be. We should be closer than ever before. But we don't talk together."

"It's just that I get very depressed by my illness," John said. "I sometimes feel my family would be better off if I were gone and it were over with. They wouldn't be burdened with me any longer—particularly Sue."

"We don't feel that way," Sue said firmly.

John persisted. "But I feel that way."

"So he withdraws into himself and doesn't communicate."

"I realize I keep too much to myself."

"We used to talk freely. There was a warmth."

"I think we still do."

"Much less."

I broke the ensuing silence. "John, do you feel that by talking about it, you just add to their burden?"

"It's not that. I don't like to talk about my illness. I look ill. I feel ill. There's all this sickness in the house. Why in the world should I carry on? What's there to be gained? I'm not enjoying life."

Sue interrupted, "Dr. Rosenbaum thinks this extended time should be lived. Your attitude can help you to live it."

John turned toward us. "But what if you're not capable of living it?"

Toward the end of July John had another remission from his cancer as a result of taking BCG and chemotherapy. His neck masses were again reduced in size, although he felt sick and weak intermittently. Then in August the flu-like symptoms from the BCG recurred. But however much John was suffering physically, I was still convinced that depression was playing a role in depriving him of any possibility of enjoyment. John agreed. One afternoon toward the end of August he commented, "The last couple of months have been the worst I've ever put in. I feel so weak all the time. I'm beginning to wonder whether it's cancer or nerves."

"Which do you think it is?" I asked.

"It could be nerves. We went to San Francisco to the Ice Follies on Sunday. I wasn't going to go, but I did, and I felt better. I forgot myself and found I had more strength than I realized.

"It's the normal day's routine that gets to me. I get up tired. I go to bed tired. I come home tired. I work five hours a day, from eight to eleven in the morning—and I find I can barely make it till eleven— when I come home and have some pudding and half-and-half to settle my stomach. I rest before having a bite of lunch, although I don't eat much. Then I go back to work at one o'clock and by three I'm ready to come home again. At that time I have a 7-Up float and sleep until six. When dinner's over, I go back to bed, usually around eight o'clock. And it's the same routine day in and day out.

"That's why I'm continually wondering whether I'm doing the right thing taking chemotherapy. As you know, my last surgeon told me, 'You'll just be sick continually and it won't do you one bit of good.' Well, I am sick a good deal of the time, and I'm of no use at home or in the office, even though my employers are kind enough to pay me. I freely admit I've thought of suicide many times. But at least I should probably stop chemotherapy and let nature take its course."

"Yet you agree that chemotherapy isn't causing all your problems," I reminded him.

"I don't think the actual process of chemotherapy is doing it. I think it's the fear of it, and the anticipation, and not knowing what's going to happen. I need to have everything cut and dried ahead of me. Yesterday I went out and bought a funeral plot. I plan ahead."

"So there it is. He's planning for death," Sue blurted out.

But I could not agree. "Most of us just ignore the fact that some-day we're going to die. I think you were right to make those arrange-ments. It takes a lot of courage not to leave it to someone else. But now you've taken care of that, and from now on I think that concentrating too much on death in the unpredictable future can defeat you in the present. Is there any way you can think of to approach the present differently, to try to counteract some of the depression?"

"I don't know how to counteract it."

"It's a vicious circle," Sue added.

"How do you feel about living in the present, Sue?" I asked.

"Well, I feel that if he only has six months, I'd rather live those six months. I'm in it as much as he is because we're living together. And yet I can't expect him to go beyond his physical capabilities. But within those capabilities we should do things together and enjoy the time we have."

"It would be nice if you could get away for weekends," I suggested.

"We were going to go away this weekend, but John panicked and we had to cancel."

John explained, "I didn't think I could eat out in restaurants for two or three days."

I did not think John should "let nature take its course," but I could appreciate his desire for some respite from chemotherapy. Lately he had suffered the side effects without experiencing the benefits of treatment. We discussed the matter at length and agreed to eliminate chemotherapy treatments for the month of September.

"All we'll do is take some X rays and carefully watch your case," I said. "It'll give you a rest and a chance to regain your equilibrium. We haven't kidded each other, John. You're in trouble."

John looked out the window. "That's something that's always bothered me. Am I going to make it this year? Am I going to make it next year?"

"I hope you're going to make it this year. Your troubles may well stabilize. Next year is a question mark. I hope to get you through this year in halfway decent shape."

"Like I am today?"

"Yes. I also hope you'll get those reservations back and have a nice weekend. Even if you can't enjoy your meals, you can still relax and walk in the woods."

"You're right. I always worry about something before it happens. I'm high-strung."

"That's true," Sue affirmed. "Even before cancer, he was this type of person."

I said, "Cancer just magnifies your problems—the ones you've had all your life. They become accentuated under stress."

Sue and John got their reservations back and then had to cancel again. Despair and cancer had effectively incapacitated John and he now began to deteriorate rapidly. His neck nodules grew, his liver became enlarged, and his pain was persistent. Even then he continued to work several hours a day. He was anxious to complete the year's work for financial reasons. "At the end of December I get a commission on the year's sales, and our sales were good this year. Money is important to me. After all, that's what I'm working for. We use everything we have on two incomes."

In mid-September John and I discussed his medical alternatives. They were limited. He had been through all the major chemotherapeutic regimens, and unless a new one was developed, any further treatment would only be detrimental. However, there was one possibility. "There is a new drug you might try," I told him, "although it's not specifically for melanoma. It's simple and nontoxic, so if you get sick, it won't be the drug. All you have to do is take three capsules a day at home."

John began taking the new drug in early October, but other problems intervened. Intense pain in a lesion in his hip brought him to the hospital in the middle of the month. I told him we would try to relieve the pain with local radiation. "Melanoma is an odd thing. It can be sensitive or insensitive to radiation. You can't tell ahead of time. But you're in a pain pattern right now and our job is to get you some relief or to break the pattern altogether. Sometimes I've knocked people out for a whole day with complete sedation and analgesia and broken the pattern."

"How long will I be out of work?" was John's natural response.

"If we have success with radiation, you should get pain relief between seven and twenty-one days, but you may be too fatigued to return to work immediately. Our job now is to get you through this acute phase."

We talked some more about medication and other details, but before leaving his room, I asked, "John, during the intervals these last weeks and months when you had some relief from pain and nausea, did you experience any happiness at all, or has it been one struggle day after day?"

The sadness in his eyes reminded me of that first day in my office. "It's been one struggle day after day. There have been no good days, really—not in the last two months."

I was regretful. "What bothers me is, we've made all these moves to give you a better quality of life. But there is no way to prophesy the results of treatment. One can only treat, wait, and hope. And we still hope to knock down your present pain so that you can be comfortable."

By the end of October John was despondent. The radiation was not completely effective in reducing his pain, which meant that he was partly dependent on narcotics. Surgery was not a possibility; the available regimens of chemotherapy and immunotherapy had been exhausted. X rays showed that the nodules in his lungs had grown and that his melanoma had spread to his brain.

Sue and the children were traveling two hours each day to visit John, as were other close relatives and friends. At that time our only medical option was to keep John comfortably sedated, so we agreed with his family that it would be best to return him to his hometown hospital. However, before making the transfer, John asked, "Is it going to come slowly, or is it going to come quickly? The only thing I worry about and fear is going out slowly with all this pain and mental anguish for myself and my family. If I suffer, my family suffers."

I reassured him he would not suffer, adding, "I've talked to the doctors who will be in charge at your local hospital and they're very capable. Also, you know I'll always be available for consultation."

John died two weeks later, in his hometown hospital, with as much pain relief and comfort as his doctors could administer.

When I look back at John's experience with cancer, my admiration for him increases. His case is an example of the frustrations that can arise for both patient and physician. Here was a man whose character was shaped by a youth of poverty, of early and endless work, who in adulthood was to find his deepest satisfactions in hard work. It was the means by which he expressed love and achieved self-esteem. When his disease progressed and therapy failed, I wanted to give him hope, but I could not combat his feeling of worthlessness when he was unable to work.

John suffered many of the worst potential problems that may arise for a cancer patient—the failure of early detection, the insensitivity of two of his doctors, his predisposition against treatment, and medical failure after the achievement of initial control through immunotherapy and chemotherapy. If chemotherapy had been more successful for a longer period, perhaps John's attitude toward therapy would have been more positive. Yet in retrospect I would still advocate therapy for John because one never knows who may respond, or when. I continue to give new patients the advice I gave John that first day in my office, "You can't quit until you've tried."

And John did try. Sue recently told me, "In September of 1972, when John was informed that his melanoma had spread to his liver and lungs, it was the first time he knew he couldn't lick it. He gathered us together in the living room and explained that all he could gain was time. Even then, although he later had moments of being morose because of the inconvenience, side effects, and eventually the futility, of treatment, he never really lost heart until the last few weeks of his life." And when I asked Sue to assess the value of treatment, she said, "It was worth it for John and it was worth it for his family. We had him four years. We might have had him for only two."

9 · Elisabeth Lee

I've never been one of those women who runs around buying lots of clothes and having her hair done. I'm neither young, nor the world's most beautiful woman, but I liked my body and wanted to have all the pieces. I'll never quite accept the loss of my breasts.

What happened to me is a little different from what happens to most women who develop breast cancer. Fifteen years ago I had a biopsy for cysts in my breasts. The test results were negative, but after that the doctors watched me closely. Other cysts developed and disappeared. Then two years ago, in April 1973, my gynecologist ordered a xeromammogram because I had a new cyst in each breast. Nothing showed up in the test results. Nevertheless, after further consultation the doctors agreed that I shouldn't take any chances and that biopsies of the cysts should be performed.

I agreed to have the biopsies but I was in an utter panic. This is the first part of the emotional crisis for a woman in whom cancer of the breast is suspected. She continuously wonders whether she'll emerge from the operation with both breasts, one breast, or no breasts. Moreover, I was, and still am, very frightened of the effects of anesthesia.

To my great relief, when I awoke from the operation I still had both breasts. The lumps had been benign.

Then a month later, when I went to see my surgeon for a checkup of the biopsy incisions, he told me that although the cysts had been benign, the cells around one of the cysts were beginning to change. He wanted to remove that breast. He said he hadn't told me before because he wanted to be certain beforehand. He wanted additional consultative opinions on the biopsies. However, I wish I had known he was thinking about it because I would have had time to prepare myself. I'm the kind of person who would rather know. I need time. I think I could accept almost anything if I just had time to think it through carefully.

The first thing I did was telephone my husband, who was on

a business trip. He became more upset than I did because he knew I was upset. He's a very concerned and sensitive man.

I couldn't believe it was happening to me. I was terrified. I had been born late in my parents' life and was consequently exposed to some fairly Victorian attitudes, one of which was my mother's belief that the removal of a breast is the worst thing that can happen to a woman. I now know it isn't the worst thing, but I thought it was at the time and told the doctor how I felt. He said most women feel the same way, that they'd rather he took out inches or feet of intestine than go near a breast.

What made my case unusual was that the cells in question showed only local and early changes. They were becoming malignant, but there was a 65-percent chance that the tumor might never progress. Such early detection is rare, and I felt that I had an option to do nothing. However, my surgeon didn't agree. He said it was the ideal time to operate, and that it would be suicide not to have it done as soon as possible. He felt that when a person has a 30- to 35-percent chance of getting cancer, and a nearly 100-percent chance of prevention and cure by surgery, there should be no question as to the course to follow. He gave me two weeks to think it over, and I told him that during that interval I wanted to talk to other doctors. I explained that it wasn't a lack of faith in him. I just didn't want to have any regrets. I wanted to be positive that it really had to be done. What if someone along the line had made a mistake? He wasn't offended.

I consulted several doctors, one of whom was a close friend. This doctor also sympathized with my need for certainty and arranged a consultation with Dr. Rosenbaum, who recommended that I have both breasts removed at the same time. He said that my breast tumor was uncommon and that because of its particular pathology there was approximately a 25-percent chance that the same process was occurring in the other breast.

I also consulted other women who had had mastectomies, but I was very careful whom I chose. I sought out women who seemed to have common sense because some people become very emotional and tend to say such things as "You must do this" and "You mustn't do that." One friend who had had a radical mastectomy several months earlier said simply, "It's not the kind of thing you want. It's the kind of thing you accept and live with."

There were many considerations. I have three children, who were then eleven, thirteen, and fifteen. I wondered what would happen to them if I didn't have the operation and I died. And if I did have the operation, how would that affect my relationship with my husband? Would he still want to go to bed with me? Could I let him go to bed with me? The doctors assured me that a marriage that is solid doesn't suffer from the removal of one breast or two breasts, but I wasn't so sure. I told my husband that if I lost my

breast I'd never again go to bed with him. He said, "That's rub-
bish. I love you and it makes no difference to me." I still couldn't
believe it wouldn't change our relationship. We discussed the fact
that losing a breast is equivalent to a man's losing his testicles.
Telling him all my apprehensions was a great relief.

As the results came in from the doctors I consulted, I became
more and more convinced that the operation was necessary. Their
opinions were unanimous. Nevertheless, I needed that period of
time for reflection.

There was one other doctor who helped me. He said he had had
a patient who was faced with a decision similar to mine. She told
the doctor she would think it over and talk to her husband about
it. Then she phoned him a week later and announced that she
would prefer to die with her body intact. The doctor persisted and
suggested she think it over, but she never called back. She died.

I decided to have one breast removed. I think that if I had had
another week to decide, or if I had been able to talk to just one
woman who had had both breasts removed at the same time, I
might have chosen to have a double mastectomy.

My husband was very supportive. I know that some husbands
aren't, and that would be the end as far as I'm concerned. We
decided not to tell our eleven-year-old the full details because we
felt he was too young, but we told the older two. They were very
frightened, especially our thirteen-year-old boy. When Dr. Rosenbaum was told about their reactions, he invited the four of us to his
office and explained everything to the children. He treated them
as adults, presenting my case exactly as it had developed and ex-
plaining the rationale for surgery. He told them where they could
obtain reading material, if they wanted to, and encouraged them
to ask questions. After an hour of discussion, they accepted it very
well, which was an enormous relief to me. If a mother knows her
children aren't upset, it helps her to get through her ordeal.

Fortunately, my mother lives with us, so there was someone
available to take care of the children. The temporary absence of
a mother must be a tremendous burden in families where no extra
help is available. Of course, relatives and friends do step in, but I
think these are problems that doctors don't always have time to
consider.

The night before the operation my surgeon visited me and talked
with my husband and me. He was very kind. My husband had previously asked him and Dr. Rosenbaum whether it might not be
possible to remove only the inside of the breast and leave the
shell and the nipple. We had heard of cases where this was done
and silicone implanted later. This was therefore considered in the
plan, although the surgeon warned us that if anything more was
found during the operation, it would be necessary to perform a
radical mastectomy.

The possibility that they might leave the shell was a great help to me psychologically. But I also seemed to have lived through certain emotions. When I went to the hospital for the biopsy six weeks earlier, I had been very frightened, and when the possibility of the mastectomy was first mentioned, I was in an utter panic, a quiet panic but an all-engulfing one. Now I was reasonably calm. Since that time I have talked to others and am convinced that most people go through similar sequences of emotion.

It proved possible to keep the shell of my breast, although I began to wonder whether they'd really found all the troublesome cells. I thought, "Perhaps they missed a couple. Maybe I'm going to die of breast cancer anyway and needn't have gone through all this." Then I pushed all that to the back of my mind and put my faith in the doctors, and in God.

Suddenly it was time to go home and begin my real adjustment. I discussed my feelings openly with my family, the doctors, and a few close friends, but I knew it would be hard for me if many people knew; and it's amazing how you can do all this without anyone's finding out. I suppose I didn't want people to know because I'm a perfectionist and this made me less than perfect. Some people want everyone to know. I feel that what happens to my body is a private matter.

Through some oversight, I was never given any information about prosthetic devices, although I now know the American Cancer Society's Reach to Recovery Program* provides all kinds of valuable information, not only about the different textures of prosthetic devices and where to buy them, but about special bathing suits, other sport clothes, and nightgowns for women who've had mastectomies. So there I was, on my way out to dinner one evening, and flat on one side. First I tried cotton, then Kleenex. All of us pushed it around to see how it looked. The children knew it was serious but they joked about it too, and that was something that really helped me.

The next day I phoned some stores and found I could buy devices that ranged from a dollar to seventy dollars. I settled on the one-dollar item. I was lucky to have enough tissue left to keep my bra from riding up, because not being able to keep a bra in place can be a real problem for a woman, psychologically and practically. A suction device that really works is quite expensive. However, a plastic surgeon told me that even when women must have the entire breast removed, he can still put a little something there to provide some bulk.

I have painful memories too. I thought I'd never take a bath again. I just didn't want to look at myself. I used to run around the house with no clothes on and my children would come in

* See Chapters 16 and 17.

and talk to me while I was taking a bath. Now I locked the bathroom door. I wouldn't even let my husband see me without clothes, and I still make love with my nightgown on. I felt my husband didn't deserve all this. After all, in our culture foreplay usually begins with the breast, and I felt, "Why does he have to have someone who's mutilated when there are other women in the world?" I'm a somewhat insecure person, and this brought out many of my insecurities.

I told Dr. Rosenbaum how I felt, and we had a long, frank talk about the realities of my situation, my marriage, and my attitude toward my body and sexual relations. He suggested I see a psychiatrist, and I did speak to one several times. He helped me a great deal, although I still find it hard to relate to my husband in bed as well as I did before. I know it's my fault and that it's all in my head, but it's still difficult.

Luckily, I didn't have a lot of time to worry after the operation. I'm in a position where I can be very helpful to my husband in his work. I've always been involved in doing things for him and the children. One of them was graduating from junior high school and another was preparing to go away for the summer, so fortunately I was busier than usual.

The summer passed quickly, and on the advice of Dr. Rosenbaum, but with the surgeon's reluctant approval, I entered the hospital in October 1973 to have my other breast removed. Just before the operation I again began to have second thoughts. Dr. Rosenbaum visited me, and after a supportive talk I mustered the courage to remain for the second surgery. As suspected, the results of the operation showed multiple areas of early cancer in the other breast.

It is now March 1975 and I still have not had the silicone implants. The surgeon wanted me to wait six months after the removal of the second breast. He said it was for reasons of infection, but I think he wanted to be sure nothing recurred, which was fine with me because that was one of my first concerns regarding implants. If something occurs under the implant, how will they find it? I also wonder whether it's wise to put foreign substances in your body, although Dr. Rosenbaum tells me the silicone is actually inside a plastic bag. It's like a Baggie with the proper shape, so there are no strange substances seeping into your system.

There is another problem. They tell me that because of the way they had to perform the operations on my breasts, one side may not look as good as the other after the implants are made. They may have to do that side twice. At least it can be done under local anesthetic, which removes one of my greatest fears.

I'm still considering the possibility of reconstruction, although my condition doesn't bother me the way it once did. Dr. Rosenbaum feels that if I can reduce the amount of disfigurement it's worth my having the implants. He has told me I won't be the same as before, but he thinks I might get some emotional satisfaction from having them. As far as the shells are concerned, I have no feeling in one side, but some feeling is beginning to return to the skin and nipple on the other side. That may be unusual, as I was told not to expect any feeling. I think surgeons prefer to be cautious in predicting the results of an operation because each case is so different.

On the plus side, I know I have every chance for a complete cure because my cancer was caught before it really got started. If I'd waited five or ten years, it might have been a different story. I'm grateful it's over and that there were doctors who were wise enough to pursue an elusive problem and find out what the trouble was. I'm thankful it was operative because there are many people who can't have surgery or who have a cancer in an area where early detection is difficult.

I was lucky in many other ways. I had a loving, supportive husband and children who needed me. It would have been harder if I had been twenty-one years old and had never had children. It would have been harder if my children had already grown up and gone away. I didn't have to worry about expense, which was more than it might have been because I had the separate operations. Even though we have good insurance, there's a great deal that's not covered. I also had enough money to consult a psychiatrist. This is a luxury when the main problem is medical, but it's just as important.

If I have undergone any other psychological changes than the ones I've described, I think I've developed a greater feeling of responsibility for others. When doctors have given their skill to save you, you feel it is incumbent upon you to do something with your life. When you look back over the years, the most important thing will be what you've done to help people. Although I'm still involved with my family's activities, I try to find more time to help other people. I especially want to help women who are faced with the alternatives I was faced with. I would first urge them to overcome their fear of going to the doctor; and I would urge them not to postpone surgery, if it is recommended. They will experience the same stages of fear, disbelief, and acceptance that I did. They will be devastated at first, but they will find that as they cope successfully with each stage of fright and denial, they will slowly build the emotional strength that will see them through their ordeal. After a while the feelings of devastation and nakedness will be eased. And they will be grateful, as I am, to be alive.

Part IV
The Family

A family faced with the life-threatening illness of one of its members has the dual problem of trying to control its own fear and anxiety while giving encouragement and support to the patient. This is just the first of many dichotomies that can arise between inner feelings and outward behavior. It can produce a situation in which members of the family and friends spend their time wondering how to ease the emotional suffering of the patient while the patient is busy worrying about the despair of those he loves. Each of them is searching for the most tactful way to deal with the other. In this search they may consider trying a candid approach but reject that option as potentially devastating. I am convinced, however, that a deliberate policy of candor and openness will create an atmosphere that is beneficial to all concerned.

Living with Cancer is based on my belief that candor creates confidence and trust between a doctor and the patient and his family. Candor between a patient and his family can achieve similar results by removing the burden of secrecy and opening the door for the alleviation of apprehensions. Candor is not easily achieved. Some people are not in the habit of speaking of their deepest concerns. Even those who have established a close relationship may become fainthearted in the presence of cancer and the threat of death. To achieve openness and to maintain it under stress is part of the challenge of living with cancer.

As a doctor I think I can be a catalyst in helping a family establish open communication about cancer and the terrors it evokes. In the early chapters of this book I described how I try to initiate a relationship based on candor by holding frank discussions with each patient and his family about the particular medical problem and its implications for their future. I emphasize the importance of asking questions and discussing problems as they arise, to forestall a more serious anxiety state. Having been brought together in this way and having experienced

101

the relief that open discussion can bring, they will, I hope, continue to relate to each other candidly about their cancer problems after they leave my office.

If they do continue such discussions in the privacy of their home, they will reap the benefits I mentioned. They need not lead a double life, hiding their real feelings while trying to guess what the other is thinking. Hearing what the other is experiencing can never be as devastating as what the imagination can conjure. Fears and frustrations can be talked about as they arise and not left to fester until they become too frightening to mention, or until a habit of withholding evolves into irretrievable isolation. The confrontation of each other's fears therefore becomes a means of keeping those fears under control. This will allow the relationship to operate in a new realm, where despair can sometimes be minimized or set aside, and enjoyment and pleasure can resume their rightful place.

Candor between a patient and his family and friends includes a recognition of each other's needs as well as fears. A family needs to give, to feel it is doing something practical to hasten the patient's recovery, whether he is at home or in the hospital.

The separation caused by hospitalization is particularly traumatic; it can cause extreme emotional distress to the members of a family. They leave the hospital each evening and worry whether their loved one will ever again lead a normal life, or whether he will even leave the hospital. Feeling impotent, they need to give of themselves. Fortunately, there are many practical services a patient's family can perform for him while he is in the hospital—services such as feeding, walking, turning, massaging. These, along with the offer of special foods, a favorite pillow, or a comforting hand, become the routine of the daily hospital visit, giving solace to family and patient alike.

When a person is critically ill, it is not unusual for at least one family member to be in attendance around the clock. This may involve sleeping in a chair beside the patient's bed or arriving early in the morning. To obtain up-to-date information on the patient's condition, relatives may rearrange their schedules so as to be present when the doctor makes his rounds or a particularly helpful nurse is on duty.

When a person is at home, functioning well, there are still many opportunities to give emotional support through practical means. One need only consider the trials a cancer patient must sometimes undergo. He may be anxious about a visit to his doctor, wondering whether a new problem will be discovered or a new treatment recommended. He may not have transportation to and from the doctor's office, or he may be dreading the side effects from the day's treatment. A spouse, parent, or friend can offer him a ride or accompany him on the bus. If family members are working and unable to be with him during the day, there is still the evening, when the side effects of therapy may have to be endured. Patient and family benefit from any means by which love and encouragement can be expressed.

To be realistic, however, not every family is able to be open, loving, or intelligently supportive, before or after a crisis. Even people who feel they have a stable relationship may find it severely threatened by the pressures of long-term illness. Latent problems may emerge. Formerly controlled anger or guilt may surface in sudden attack or recrimination, indifferent or oversolicitous behavior. Or just the exhaustion and frustration of constant worry and care may break the most loyal supporter.

Lengthy illness can also break the most courageous of patients. When a person has fought long and hard against cancer, lost and regained hope many times, and then realizes the battle is not to be won, he may at times experience rage and depression that will seek as their target the nearest available person—spouse, child, parent, or the nurse on duty. This anger is usually manifested as irritation over trivial matters that in normal times would not even concern the patient. The person under attack needs to understand that this is not a rejection of him but a cry of anguish.

In addition to anger and depression, a patient must also endure the endless boredom of being ill, as well as the fear of being a burden when he really wants and needs special attention. Ironically, the people from whom he wants this attention may be suffering from the same tedium or from feelings of inadequacy and guilt for being unable to relieve his suffering. They may not be able to cope with the reality in which the patient is imprisoned. The result may be a gradual diminishment of attention and care by the family and increased bitterness and fear of isolation in the patient.

No one should be blamed for the way he responds to the crisis of a long-term illness or the threat of change and loss. Some people and some relationships grow stronger; some waver and hold together; others collapse. I believe that those who strive toward the ideal of candor and sharing in their relationships can not only hold together but also experience new depths of love, respect, and understanding.

I have often thought it is a shame that some people have to develop a fatal disease before they realize the value of life and love, family and friends. I am not implying that just because a person has cancer a light will shine or bells ring out, or that he will become clairvoyant. This heightened appreciation may simply evolve from the common effort of patient, family, friends, and doctor to find solutions to the medical and emotional problems that cancer can bring. It is the suc-

cessful interaction of these people that contributes to mutual understanding and strengthens love. It is these experiences that give life its
worth and dignity.

Following are the stories of several patients, each of whom is unique—
in himself, in his type of cancer and medical outlook, in the availability
and willingness of family and friends to support him, and in the degree
of candor he and they allow to exist.

10 · Darrell Ansbacher

September 1973

"When Darrell feels bad, we feel bad. We let our empathy flow to him and hope that it gives him strength. Every single one of his problems is our problem, and because we share, it becomes easier to bear all around."

Mr. Ansbacher smiled at Darrell, the younger of his two sons, who was about to complete a course of radiotherapy for Hodgkin's disease. The disease had been discovered the previous June when Darrell, aged eighteen, home for the summer from his freshman year in college, had consulted his family physician about a swelling in his groin. Darrell had been confident that a shot of penicillin would dispense with the problem. However, a negative examination and blood tests alerted his physician to other possibilities and he arranged for a biopsy the following day.

It was now a warm evening in September, when summer comes to San Francisco. I had stopped at the Ansbacher home to chat with Darrell and his parents about their experiences during the past three months.

"Has Darrell's illness brought you closer together as a family?" I asked.

"People say a crisis brings a family together, but that hasn't been the case in our family," Mr. Ansbacher replied. "We've always been close. Our children have always felt they could come to us, and vice versa. Moreover, I remember when all this happened, Darrell was with his friend Roger, and Roger came out of the house and said, 'You know, Darrell is worried about you.' That's the kind of relationship we have in this family."

We then discussed the period of the diagnosis.

"I was very fortunate," said Darrell. "I know that some people can have Hodgkin's for years and not know it. A doctor who was less concerned and less skillful than our family physician might not have observed the symptoms and recommended that I have the proper tests and a biopsy.

"However, even though I was undergoing all those tests, I don't think I was really aware that it might be something serious until you told me I had a malignancy in my lymph nodes but that the possibility of leukemia had been eliminated."

Mr. Ansbacher added, "When we were told a malignancy was diagnosed, the blow was incredible. Then, as the results came in and we discovered it was Hodgkin's, and we were told what the prospects were at that stage of the game, all of a sudden I was happy with Hodgkin's. You're grateful for small favors."

His wife nodded in agreement. "The first relief was that there was a chance for a complete cure, so we were free to concentrate on the next step, which we felt had to be carried out as quickly and efficiently as possible. I think as parents our biggest comfort was our involvement in getting things done fast and well."

Events did move swiftly for the Ansbachers. In the days following Darrell's visit to his family doctor, he had a bone-marrow examination, a biopsy of the swelling in his groin, X rays of the chest, a lymphangiogram, and an intravenous pyelogram, as part of the preliminary staging of the amount of disease. When the approximate degree of Hodgkin's disease had been determined, Darrell and his parents were referred for consultation and further explanation to Dr. Henry Kaplan, a leading authority on Hodgkin's disease at Stanford University Medical School. I alerted them to the probability that he would recommend exploratory abdominal surgery, a procedure that is now almost routine in determining more precisely the extent of spread of the disease. In such exploratory surgery a biopsy of the liver and lymph nodes is performed, and the spleen removed. After early childhood, the spleen, essentially a large lymph node, is considered expendable—it has served its function of providing the body with an immune defense system (lymphocytes) while the body is developing its own system of antibodies. Thus it can be removed and examined without interfering with any natural functions. If the spleen is unaffected by Hodgkin's disease, it is almost certain that the liver is unaffected; if the spleen shows evidence of disease, then there may be liver involvement.

"I was very apprehensive about how the details were going to be conveyed to us by Dr. Kaplan," Mr. Ansbacher recalled. "Was he going to ask my wife and me to come into his office while Darrell waited outside, or would he take Darrell into his office and leave us outside? He did neither of those things. He invited us all into his office, saying, 'I'm going to tell each one of you the same thing at the same time. Nobody is going to be kept in the dark about anything.' Then he laid it on the line very bluntly, without any reservations, telling Darrell, 'You may as well forget about the next year of your life because it's going to be a very difficult year.' However, he also confirmed your reassuring statements that in Darrell's case there was an 80- to 90-percent chance for a complete cure.

"Of course since that conversation we've found the system of sharing information has worked so well that we've made a pledge to each other to continue it."

In the ten days following the original biopsy, Darrell underwent three days of tests at Mount Zion Hospital, visited Dr. Kaplan and was tested at Stanford, and entered Mount Zion on July 4 in preparation for exploratory surgery the next day.

Darrell said, "There was a party the night before I was admitted to the hospital. It was a strange experience going to this party, knowing that the next day I was admitting myself to the hospital. I was actually letting myself in for it. Nevertheless, since it was to be done, I was lucky not to have to wait to be admitted until after the holiday."

"I think a doctor should keep in mind that waiting a week, or even over a weekend, for an operation may seem normal to him, but may be an excruciating interval for a patient and his family," Mrs. Ansbacher added.

In the exploratory surgery on July 5 Darrell's spleen and appendix were removed, his lymph nodes resected, and bone marrow and liver biopsies taken. The results were pretty much as we had suspected—slight spleen and lymph-node involvement and a good chance for complete cure. However, a cure could not be effected without complete nodal radiation and a course of complementary chemotherapy.

Of the lengthy process of cure, Mr. Ansbacher commented, "We have decided to take each day as it comes. That's the only way we ourselves can cope, and we hope our attitude flows to Darrell so he can cope with it too."

"How much have these last weeks of traveling to Stanford for radiation disrupted your lives?" I inquired.

"First of all, we don't think in terms of our lives being disrupted. My wife and I have never considered that anything our children required was a sacrifice. The word 'sacrifice' never entered our vocabulary because we never thought it or felt it. What has disrupted our lives, though, is the sorrow of seeing a child agonizing and losing weight.

"We take turns driving Darrell to Stanford. My wife goes twice a week. I go once. And Richard, my older son, goes once. But we never forget that Darrell has to go four days in a row. Our only goal is to make him feel better. But when I went today, I came away feeling better for having gone. When I don't go, I don't feel so good. I also went into the radiation room with him once, just to see. I felt that way I could empathize even more with him. They explained how the various lead shields are made, how thick they are, and how Darrell was being prepared for the treatment. They gave me a feeling it was being done right—not that I'd know if it weren't. But I'd seen it. I felt better. And I think the family needs to be made to feel better too. It's a heavy burden for us."

"We've had other help, too," said his wife thoughtfully. "Do you remember the social worker who was in the radiation area the first day?" Turning to me, she explained, "She sat down and spoke briefly to all of us, telling us what was going to happen; and then when Darrell was having his treatment, she told us what the various unpleasant effects might be, such as nausea, weight loss, fatigue, diarrhea, and the loss of his hair in patches. She said there are no two patients alike. That's terribly important to know.

"We also talked about the relief to a patient of having advance knowledge of his side effects. If and when they occur, he needn't worry that something new and terrible is happening. But the social worker then said that most people tend not to ask questions, that they come into the hospital with no idea of what's wrong and don't appear very interested in finding out.

"However, I don't think it's a lack of interest," Mrs. Ansbacher continued. "Sometimes people feel that if they ask a question, the doctor will think they are questioning his medical expertise."

"I have a good example of a patient being uninformed," said Darrell. "Yesterday I was sitting in the waiting room and I heard an elderly man on the other side of the door say something like, 'I don't understand why you have to take my blood to find out how I am. You're radiating me. I had pain in my right leg and you took out my left kidney.' Then he jokingly added, 'I'm glad I didn't have a pain in my foot or you would have cut my head off.'

"When he came out I explained to him why they took his blood. I told him how the blood count gives an indication as to how efficiently the body is functioning in spite of the radiation and how imperative it is that the body maintain a certain blood count. The man obviously had cancer and didn't know it. He even had a kidney removed without being told why."

"People are also overawed by doctors and don't want to bother them," Mr. Ansbacher commented. "Yet a question that may sound silly to a doctor isn't silly to his patient. It's terribly important that I be able to ask about anything that concerns me without being ridiculed. Nothing has happened to Darrell since June 21 for which we didn't seek out an explanation."

One thing that happened to Darrell was a daily bout with nausea following his radiation treatment. I asked him if the nausea had eased up lately, and I was also curious to know what he actually experienced each day as he went into the radiation room.

"First of all," Darrell began, "it's a very odd sensation to know that all I have to do not to be sick on any given day is to skip my radiation treatment. I have to keep reminding myself that it's for my own good.

"The routine helps me. I get up at six-thirty each day that I'm scheduled for treatment, and I'm there for the first appointment at eight o'clock. I usually have to wait a few minutes in a room with other people, most of whom are worse off than I am, with no hair on their heads, beady eyes, and some burn marks on their bodies. When my turn comes, I go into a room, take off my clothes, and put on a robe. Then I enter the radiation room. I have the same room and the same technicians each time, which is really important to me because it reinforces the routine. The room, which is underground, is about four times larger than a regular X-ray room, and it's oval-shaped, with thick cement walls. The only furniture, aside from the X-ray table, consists of three work tables laden with huge lead blocks. Each patient has a set of lead blocks that is prepared specifically to his measurements and that delineates the areas to be radiated. When you lie on the X-ray table, a mesh screen apparatus constructed like a breakfast tray is placed over you, and your particular lead block is placed on top of that. Your body is marked, so the blocks are replaced accurately each time. When the technician who has set up the screen and the block leaves the room, she goes to a window about eight by four inches and pushes a button that slides the heavy door into place. The door is inside the wall: that is, when it has slid into place, nothing is visible but a flat cement wall.

"By this time you've removed your robe, of course, so there you are, naked. It's like a waiting room for—somewhere.

"There's also an odor of lead, and a high-pitched noise for as long as you're being radiated. For me it's a minute and a half, so each time I hold a countdown and think that this is one less time I'll have to be there.

"And that's it. We travel two hours each day for one and one-half minutes of treatment. Although I usually do the driving on the way down, whoever has come with me that day drives back, because the nausea begins almost immediately.

"I do everything I can to establish and maintain routine to make it easier on myself. We park in the same place each day and walk to the cafeteria, where I have a Pepsi-Cola and a doughnut. I find that helps when the nausea comes. Although I vomited after the first few treatments, I now find I can think my way out of it. I'm home by nine-thirty and lie on my bed with a container next to me, just in case. Then

I generally goof off, watching game shows and doing puzzles until I feel better later in the day.

"The reason I try to reinforce the routine is to establish a rhythm that will make the end of treatment seem to come more quickly. It's like climbing a steep hill in San Francisco. If you keep your eye on the cracks in the cement instead of on the top of the hill, you'll seem to reach your goal in less time.

"However, to answer the rest of your question, the nausea really hasn't abated. But as you know, I've always had a weak stomach, so none of us is too worried about the meaning of the nausea. As a matter of fact, my mother is apt to urge me to go to a summer school class or to visit a friend."

"True," laughed his father. "I'm much more apt to say, 'If you don't feel well, just lie around.' I've been overprotective with both our boys in that respect. When I see Darrell with an upset stomach, I haven't the heart to urge him to do something to occupy his mind, as the doctors have recommended."

Mrs. Ansbacher observed, "Yet Darrell knows that when he goes out and is active mentally, when he doesn't have the opportunity to think about himself quite as much, he feels good when he comes home. We've all had that experience. So you just wonder how far the mind involves itself with the body."

Darrell knew. "The power of the mind to ignore the body is just incredible. Sometimes it even works adversely. I can be feeling bad but go out and be active anyway, and then later find myself wishing I hadn't."

"I think Darrell's age raises a question here," said his mother. "How much do you insist that he do, and how much do you let him make up his own mind? He's been away at college and had a year of independence. He's at a crossroad. We know we have valuable experience that might be of help, but how do we get it across without sounding like a parent-child relationship? Of course, some decisions were never in our hands. If the doctors say you have to have your spleen removed, or radiation therapy, or chemotherapy, these are just not decisions. We don't tell Darrell he's got to go through these things. He's old enough to know that's what he has to do and that if we could avoid it, we would. All we can do is act on these doctors' decisions in concert with one another and share whatever comes."

Darrell offered eloquent testimony of his parents' handling of the issue of independence. "My brother and I were always given opportunities to exercise independence. We've never felt we were being overprotected for more than an hour or so. It's never been one of those 'They'll never let me do anything' kind of things. Yet I've had friends whose parents went one step too far in cutting the cord—where the kids had to leave the house. Other kids just stayed away for three or four days at a time as opposed to going home. And when they finally did leave, it was the greatest thing in their lives. I've never had that experience, nor has Richard.

"But I think that whether you're dependent on your parents or not, when you're sick, you go to them. I was like that when I was eight. I'm like that at eighteen. And I'll probably be like that when I'm twenty-eight. If I get anything that exceeds the flu, I'll call home."

"I've often told Darrell how concerned I am about people who are alone, without family or friends. That must be really crushing. How increasingly debilitating that must be when a situation is already serious," his father said.

"There are some psychologists who say a person won't get better unless he knows it's important to someone that he does get better," said Darrell. "As far as getting better goes, one thing we've never really talked about is that by having treatment I'm interrupting my life for a year instead of losing it in five or ten years. It means there's no alternative to treatment, but it also means I haven't been concerned with death."

"But we can empathize much more now with people who are really faced with an end," said Mrs. Ansbacher.

And her husband quickly confirmed this feeling. "Obviously since this has happened to us, I feel much closer to other families with problems."

I told Mr. Ansbacher I had been curious to know how his family crisis had affected his relationships with his friends.

"Many people in the last three months have told me, 'We have good thoughts for you. Our prayers are with you.' I know these people aren't going to go home and pray for Darrell Ansbacher; I don't take them literally. But these words have been a tremendous comfort to us all. I really think that people's good thoughts for you can help."

"There is something very Jewish about our situation," Darrell said. "It's the sense of strength from the community, the strength of people coming together. Our family is in a position where we've had that kind of help and comfort, mostly from fellow Jews, members of our congregation. The cards, telephone calls, gifts, and things like that have really helped."

His mother elaborated on the beliefs that underlay that strength. "It isn't a holier-than-thou attitude. It isn't a matter of belief in God per se. It's a sense of the life force. I feel man has been put on Earth with a marvelous brain to think with. When I go to services I don't necessarily pray to God. I go there to be in an atmosphere where I marvel at Creation with all its faults and to find where I fit into it.

"Cancer is where nature has gone wrong, but I still know there are scientists with brains who can think up cures. That fits in too. I have a very comfortable attitude toward life. Whatever will be will be. I'll fight for what I have to, but I have a calm attitude about when my time will come, or my husband's time will come. I have this attitude because of our religious background. I feel I have something to hold on to."

January 1974

Darrell returned to college one month late, at the end of October, upon completion of his radiation treatments. He had only six weeks in Los Angeles, free of all therapy, before coming back to San Francisco at the end of the fall quarter, in time to begin his first twenty-eight-day cycle of a six-month course of chemotherapy. The cycle consisted of an intravenous shot on the first and the eighth days of the cycle, in addition to pills taken orally on the first fourteen days. The fifteenth through twenty-eighth days were free of medication.

Darrell and I talked in my office the day after he had received his first shot of the second cycle. He planned to return to Los Angeles the next day and to commute to San Francisco on the days he was to receive his shots. I first asked him how being a month late at college had worked out for him.

"I had put a huge amount of emphasis on getting back to school at the beginning of the quarter. I'm not sure why. It wasn't that necessary, although part of it was that I had made plans with several people. I did get out of time with a lot of people but that was more because I was taking eight units and they were taking full loads. I couldn't keep up with them."

I then commented on the tremendous role his parents had played in helping him through his operation and his radiation treatments, and asked, "How did they react when you returned to school?"

"When I first left, they were both a little timid about it. They weren't sure it was the right thing to do. But now they see that I thrive in Los Angeles, so even though their first response is, 'Let's keep him at home where we can protect him,' they're happy to have me be there.

"I think a lot of my problem has been psychological, my nerves. This is probably true of everybody, but perhaps of myself a little more so. As long as I can keep my mind occupied, I think I stand a better chance of avoiding a lot of the discomfort that comes with all this. In Los Angeles I can do that. Also, my brother is in Los Angeles and I like being where he is. My parents know I'm only an hour away, and that if anything serious happens my first move will be toward the airport. Naturally the whole idea of doing everything right medically is the most important thing. Everything else is secondary."

"How do you think it's going to work out to be in Los Angeles and to commute to San Francisco for your shots? Do you think you can handle it?" I asked.

"At first I was very optimistic. I was going to take my shot, be out for a day, and then be back at work, like the stories I've heard. But after the second shot, in December, when I found I didn't have the best reaction, I became pessimistic and thought perhaps I'd spend the two weeks that I'm on chemotherapy at home, and the two weeks that I'm off down in Los Angeles. However, now I'm back on the optimistic attitude again. Tomorrow I'll return to Los Angeles and try to conduct myself as normally as possible. Because this next week, when I'll be between the two shots, is going to be a gauge for me as to how well I can handle myself when I'm feeling uncomfortable."

"I think you have a good attitude. People somehow adjust. You had more reaction initially with radiation because of fear, and that fear may be having a similar effect now that you're beginning chemotherapy. But the drug you're on does cause gastrointestinal distress in a certain percentage of people. You might help to alleviate it by nibbling small amounts of food all day long, keeping your stomach full but not eating any big meals. Then, using the antinausea medicine and changing antacids, you might try different sequences of taking your pills. Try taking both at bedtime; or try one in the morning and one in the evening. You've survived the first course and that should give you a little assurance that you can make it through the rest. It may become routine in time."

"I haven't noticed it becoming routine yet. Routine is when I know when I'm not going to feel well, and for how long, although I feel quite well considering I just had the shot yesterday."

"That's excellent. I think that shows you can tolerate it. The next question is: can you tolerate the oral pills as well? The odds are you can, and you will get whatever you need as antinausea medicine."

"Actually my apprehension has decreased a little now that the first series is over. And this has lessened my father's apprehension also. He was at least as worried as I was, if not more so. The fact that chemotherapy doesn't occur every day, as radiation did, is also a help. My body may need two weeks off between the chemicals, but my parents also need two weeks off in between my discomfort."

"Have you noticed any other changes in your feelings or attitudes? Many of my patients have said they develop a new viewpoint while living with a malignancy. It's not that their basic personalities undergo radical change, but they say they perceive themselves and their relationships more clearly. They feel calmer, more certain about the things they want to do and what they want to eliminate from their lives."

"Since I've been home for Christmas, many of my friends say I've mellowed quite a bit. I used to talk a lot. There was a laugh-a-minute way about me. I'm still the same person. I laugh at the same jokes. But I seem to take things easier. I don't know whether that's because I don't have the energy or because I've really mellowed. I am tired more often than I used to be. I sleep more and I'm sick much of the time. I look forward to when I'll be finished with therapy because it will only be then that I'll really be able to sit back and relax.

"I've changed in one respect, however. Something that would have made me very nervous before—the rent being overdue or being late for something—I find I don't worry as much about these things because I've had something in my life that was really worth worrying about. I saw my friends during this last quarter at school panic when final exams came around, especially the premeds. I don't say this to their faces, and I don't know why I don't, but I wonder what disease they're going to get before they realize what's important. I find my own grade-point average is higher because of this attitude. I take it much easier, and I think that once this is all over, it will really have made an improvement in my life."

"How else are you different, aside from this ability to take things easier and this sense of what's really important?"

"I'm a lot more timid. My daring has been cut back because I'm worried about the physical repercussions. But as time goes on, my fear of the daring has become less. What I try to do is be daring in a pattern, a little more daring each time, to build up my tolerance."

"Do your parents worry about your being too daring?"

"Yes, but I understand why they feel how they feel. When they show concern, they're just covering all the bases. When they're overprotective, I can usually convince them that they are and they ease up. They'd like —everyone would like—everything to be written down, to follow a book. It would make things much easier if a person could anticipate each thing before it happens. But since that's not possible, I understand their feelings. If we talk to each other, we can usually find a point in between where we can understand each other.

"I even think my being in Los Angeles helps them. As long as I'm around, they feel a necessity to be overprotective. When I'm away, they forget about me for a while. Even then they call every other day to find out how I'm feeling, and they know my brother is there to keep tabs on me."

Darrell and I had talked before about the book I was writing for cancer patients and their families, and I asked him now if he thought such a book would have helped him.

"I don't think it would have helped me personally because I've had my parents and my brother. I've had other things to lean on. But I think for most people that may not be the case. The strong family tie is an oddity these days."

"Is there anything special that you would tell other people who have Hodgkin's, or a lung or a stomach problem—anything that's a threat to their existence, immediately or in the distant future?"

Darrell thought for a moment. "I'm offering the point of view of someone who's on the homestretch, who has a chance of cure—and I'm speaking as a nineteen-year-old—but my advice to anyone who is considering treatment is that there is nothing they can do to you that if it saves your life will be too high a price.

"As long as you have time, as long as you have the gift of a normal life ahead of you, there is nothing you can do wrong that you can't try to undo. Perhaps one of the worst things that could happen is that you couldn't undo something you'd done.

"Time is something man invented somewhere along the line, and it really is in some ways one of the greatest inventions; in other ways it's the scariest. It gives you a beginning and an end. If there's a chance of that end being premature, there is no gamble too great to get rid of your disease. You don't worry about whether the cure will be worth it."

"What is your feeling about death at this point in your illness?"

"Not to fear death now would be a mistake, after what I've gone through to hold on to life. But I don't think my fear lies in the childish fear of death, in fear of the unknown or of darkness or being alone. It's different. I've paid the price. It's like paying an exorbitant price for a piece of jewelry and then not getting the jewelry. That's my fear now. It's as though I don't deserve death now. I've bought from the devil. I've bought time."

"I understand. You want your deserts. You want to find your happiness."

"I'm not expecting immortality or anything. I expect comfort. I want a break. It isn't as if I haven't earned it."

"You've earned it," I confirmed.

"However, there's something still in me. It isn't disease. It's something that says, 'It isn't over yet.' Lately I've indulged in a lot of daydreams of you saying, 'I bet you never thought this would be over.' And it flows out of your mouth so easily. Each time I go to your office I expect to hear those words. Unfortunately, they haven't come out yet. I'm still waiting. I know the day will come."

"You've made your contract," I assured him, "and you're going to win."

December 1974

After our conversation in January Darrell returned to Los Angeles and remained there until the end of the quarter, in early April, returning to San Francisco for a couple of days at a time to receive his shots. Although he functioned very well, despite some discomfort, he decided to skip the last quarter and to complete his chemotherapy at home in San Francisco. He told me, "School was a big thing in the beginning. I wanted to prove I could function, but that became less important as it became obvious that chemotherapy was something very debilitating."

Chemotherapy was completed by the end of May. Darrell remained at home over the summer, working part time, and returned to college in the fall, in good physical condition but aware that he was particularly susceptible to infections because of his Hodgkin's disease and his therapy.

The fall quarter went well, and when Darrell came home for the holidays we had several talks. Of the year from late June 1973 to the summer of 1974 Darrell said, "It was like having the flu for a year, a bad case of the flu.

"I could tolerate the radiation, but when it was time for the chemotherapy I actually dreaded it. I didn't have the strength to be nervous. I just didn't want to do it. I had been sure there was going to be a way out of it, but there wasn't. That intravenous stuff just blows you out. I didn't realize how debilitating it was going to be, even though you gave me all kinds of sedatives to minimize my psychological reactions. I'm still not up from it, although the nervous twitches and all the nervous energy is back."

"Yes," I said, "but you are slowly getting back your strength."

"I could be, but I haven't done the exercises. It's easy to say you want to go on a regular daily exercising routine, another thing to do it. Actually, I'd like to be playing basketball."

"Can you tell me about your nervousness and your anxiety?" I inquired.

"Yes. I wonder why things aren't different now. I have damned good reason for them to be drastically changed, and they're not. I wonder why I'm still able to drink an occasional drink or smoke an occasional cigarette when I know the farfetched possibilities of what could happen to me, just like anybody else. How come I eat food with preservatives in them? How come I'm not a health nut?

"Other things haven't changed either. I thought the whole time I was taking chemotherapy, 'Boy when this is over, those petty little things just aren't going to bother me.' That's true to a certain extent, but it's also true that when you get better again, you have the same anxieties and the same problems as before. You still have to cope with them. Disease in many ways is a way around coping with a lot of your normal problems, your inadequacies and insecurities. As long as you're sick, you can forget about them because, of course, the reason for them is that you're sick. When you're well, they'll be gone.

"I now think my so-called mellowness was a physical thing, fatigue. I think of it sometimes in terms of Scrooge. Did you ever think about what happened to Scrooge after his conversion? Did he stay the great sweet guy he became that night, or did he gradually fall back into his old pattern of being a schmuck? What happened to me was more in terms of mental anguish than what happened to Scrooge, yet I've experienced no outrageous changes. I'm still what I was before, with the same weaknesses."

"How do your parents feel, now that the ordeal is over? Do you worry about them?"

"They're not free of concern, and that does worry me. There's no way I can satisfy their need to have me around. Yet they're not stifling in any way. I'll be going back to school in four or five days, but I'm aware that my departure is more of a trauma than for any of my friends and their parents because of what we've been through. It's made a difference. Most people who say good-by are sad, and say something like 'See you in two months,' but with me I sense there's something more."

"Is it hard for you, knowing your parents are so concerned?"

"Only in that I have always tried to control my own reactions. For instance, regardless of how rotten I've ever felt, I would still say, "Well, it was worse three weeks ago,' or 'It'll be over in a little while.' Simply, that was easier. I can avoid the emotional aspects within myself. It's harder to handle when I see emotion in other people, and hardest of all when I see it in my parents. I'm not shocked or surprised. I just don't know what to do and it makes me uncomfortable.

"I've always felt this is supposed to be hard on me; there's nothing I can do about that. But if there is ever anything I can do that will make it easier for my parents, then I have no qualms about it."

"Are you doing that now?"

"Yes. I keep a lot of my feelings of nervousness from them because I feel it's best for them that they think everything is great. It does me no good for them to think otherwise. It would just be another burden for me if I knew they were worried."

"That may be the only disadvantage to having such a close family," I said.

11 · Magdalena Matunan

Magdalena and Teofilo Matunan were married in 1934 in the Philippines. In 1945 they emigrated to the United States with their three daughters and one son. They settled, with other Filipino immigrants, on a section of land on the southern perimeter of San Francisco, close to the Bay. There they raised their children, worked hard, and saved enough money to buy their own home in the same section of town, close to their friends, in 1952. Their eldest daughter, Kate, was then seventeen years old.

Kate is now forty, herself the mother of a seventeen-year-old girl and an eighteen-year-old boy. She smiles happily as she speaks of the years she and her sisters and brother spent in their parents' home. "The house was always full of people, and we always had pets. My parents shared the household chores because they were both working. Since my father liked to cook, my mother cleaned and did a lot of other things. She was never still for a minute. And she had a green thumb. I remember the windows were always full of African violets. My mother and father even fixed up an apartment for my husband, David, and me when we were first married. We lived with them for two years, until we could afford our own place and I became pregnant."

Victoria and Dely, Kate's younger sisters, are now also married, and each has three children. Victoria lives in Denver; Dely and Kate live within twenty miles of their old home. Their brother, Manuel, died when he was twelve years old.

When their children married and moved away, Magdalena and Teofilo did not seek smaller quarters. Their house remained a center of activity, a source of delight to their eight grandchildren and themselves. They also enjoyed visiting the homes of their daughters. Because they both worked—Teofilo at night and Magdalena in the daytime— these visits were limited to weekends, when they would drive about in their car, visit the grave of their son, and stop at their daughters' homes to talk and to play with their grandchildren. The three generations were in close touch.

The first hint of cancer occurred in June 1969, when Magdalena Matunan wàs fifty-four years old. Malignant cells were discovered in her right ovary, and she immediately had a hysterectomy. However, her cancer had been diagnosed early and her doctors decided against giving follow-up radiation therapy. Instead, she took hormones to replace those that her ovaries had once produced, and received a thorough checkup every six months. Life continued as before for Magdalena and Teofilo.

Then in early June 1972 Magdalena noticed a swelling in the lymph nodes in her neck. Although they gave her no discomfort, she quickly notified her doctor. A biopsy of one of the nodes revealed that Magdalena's ovarian cancer had spread to her lymph nodes on the left side of her neck, but there was no evidence of disease in her pelvis or elsewhere.

Magdalena was given local radiation on her neck for a period of five weeks. When this therapy was completed in the first week of August, the mass had been reduced. For the next four and a half months her doctors closely watched her condition but were unable to discern any other evidence of recurrence. As a precaution they talked with me in November about the advisability of putting Magdalena on a program of chemotherapy. After studying her case, I felt we must be guarded in giving a long-term prognosis because her disease had recurred so far from its point of origin. But since she was otherwise in good health, had lost little weight, and showed no evidence of liver or lung involvement, I considered her a good candidate for chemotherapy.

Magdalena began a course of chemotherapy on December 24, 1972, five days after a palpable node appeared just above the area that had been treated by radiation the previous summer. She received her chemotherapy intravenously at first, and later in tablet form. In addition to the swelling that had returned to the neck area, she had edema in her right leg, so I also prescribed a low salt diet and diuretics.

During January and February 1973, chemotherapy was successful in shrinking Magdalena's nodes, although by the end of March, with the completion of that particular chemotherapeutic program, it appeared that the neck mass was again increasing. There was also evidence of fluid in her abdomen and continuing edema in her right leg. In addition, her white blood cell count had dropped, making it necessary to wait until the count returned to a safer level before continuing with a second round of chemotherapy.

Magdalena's blood count was taken every Monday and Thursday, and toward the end of April radiotherapy was again prescribed. Her nodes were increasing in size, and her edema was worse, making her right thigh swollen and painful, and walking difficult. The second course of radiation therapy was completed on May 9, 1973, and a new round of chemotherapy begun shortly thereafter. Both legs were now afflicted with edema.

On June 20, with increasing evidence of disease in her neck and abdomen, and increased edema in her right leg, Magdalena was put on a new chemotherapeutic program. By June 29, I noted on her record, "Chances for improvement or control do not appear good."

Magdalena was one of the 50 percent of women with ovarian cancer whose disease fails to respond to chemotherapy, a tragedy for her and Teofilo and the rest of the family. I have, of course, seen many similar cases, and I have observed the ways in which families come together in support of a stricken member. However, the care that Magdalena now received from her family, particularly Teofilo, and the love and sensitivity shown to both Magdalena and Teofilo by their daughters, sons-in-law, and grandchildren, will always be a vivid and touching memory for me.

Magdalena knew what was happening to her. She asked me many times how bad things were, and I always gave her a frank reply. But she rarely discussed her prognosis with her family. One of the rare occasions when she did refer to her impending death occurred just before Christmas 1972. At her parents' home Kate was helping her mother trim the Christmas tree when her mother suddenly said, "If anything happens to me, promise me that your dad can stay with you and David." Kate's first reaction was to tell her mother not to talk that way; then she quickly reassured her that Teofilo was always welcome in her home. Magdalena concluded the conversation, saying, "I don't want your dad to stay here by himself."

In July, Magdalena was finding it increasingly difficult to walk, and in early August, when she could no longer stand by herself, Teofilo retired from his job prematurely to take care of her. I told him Magdalena's prospects for long-term survival were poor, but how much he suppressed, or how much he admitted to himself, was difficult to ascertain. His task was to take care of Magdalena, pray for a miracle, and offer constant encouragement. They had their own silent ways of helping each other.

Magdalena could just make it to the car with Teofilo's help, and during the early part of August she would urge him to take her for rides. They always followed their familiar path, visiting their son's grave before going to Kate's or Dely's home, except that these days the girls and their families would come out to the car to chat with Magdalena.

By the middle of August Magdalena could no longer go out in the car. She couldn't even get out of bed. However, Teofilo was determined that she not be hospitalized; and when a family feels this way, I always try to treat the patient at home.

Teofilo took over the management of the house. He cooked food that would please Magdalena and kept the house spotless because she liked it that way. He slept on a cot beside her bed and awakened when she did. Yet during all this time he avoided discussing Magdalena's condition with his daughters and sons-in-law. They, of course, knew without being told that Magdalena was dying, but they could not guess what Teofilo was thinking. Was he protecting himself or Magdalena or his daughters with his silence?

Kate and her sisters agreed among themselves that by preparing himself in advance, Teofilo might find it easier to face Magdalena's death when it occurred, but they were wary of broaching the subject with him. Then Kate decided that I might be the best means of approach to their father. She phoned me one afternoon and first confirmed what she already knew by asking me whether her mother was dying. The truth was shocking, nevertheless. She then spoke to me of the family's concern for Teofilo and arranged that I make a house call at an hour when she and her sisters would be together at her parents' home.

A few days later, at the appointed hour, I went to the Matunan house. After a long talk with Magdalena, I stopped in the living room, where Teofilo was sitting with his daughters. As though for the first time, Kate quizzed me about her mother's condition. I tried to respond clearly and candidly. Teofilo listened, but Kate thinks he still did not accept his wife's impending death.

Kate and her sisters visited their mother daily, and helped their father, but he remained in charge of Magdalena's care. His daughters, in turn, tried to care for him. They brought him food because he cooked only for Magdalena. They arranged that one grandchild always be present as company for Teofilo. Kate's son, Sam, said, "I come here a lot and stay with my grandfather. It's natural for us to be sad and sympathetic. Just knowing we're here helps him."

When Magdalena needed a shot, the family even had its own supply of nurses. One was a cousin who worked in a San Francisco hospital, the other a sister-in-law of Kate's husband. When it was necessary to tap the fluid in Magdalena's abdomen, I always did it at home, because home was where she wanted to be.

Magdalena and Teofilo were Catholics who had been married in a civil ceremony. Again, with no more than the breath of a wish from Magdalena, a priest was summoned and Magdalena's brothers and sisters (all of whom had immigrated to the United States) were invited to the Matunan home. In early September, in the presence of all her relatives, Magdalena was married to Teofilo in a religious ceremony. Kate recalls, "It was like a party. My mother would beckon to her brothers and sisters, one at a time. She remembered everything they did as youngsters. She'd recall funny stories with each one."

Two weeks after the wedding, Kate remembers, her mother couldn't keep her eyes open. "When we saw she was resting, we'd leave her alone. When her eyes were open and she felt like talking, we'd talk. Sometimes I'd just sit there and hold her hands and pray.

"At other times she'd be her old stubborn self, and that was wonderful. It meant she was still alert. We'd be whispering in the kitchen about what to give her for lunch, and she'd suddenly say very loudly, 'I don't *want* chicken soup.'"

Magdalena's sons-in-law were as supportive and eager to help as their wives. Victoria's husband, Larry, who had recently been ill himself, drove West from Denver on his vacation to be with Magdalena. He said, "That's what families are for and I was never close to mine." Although Dely's husband, Jim, had just started his own business, he gave all his free time to Magdalena and Teofilo with the simple explanation, "When a person is ill, people should be there." Kate and David were quietly preparing a section of their home so that Teofilo might move in when Magdalena died. These silent acts of love were instinctive, the result of years of being together and enjoying each other.

The weaker Magdalena became, the more she needed Teofilo. He sat with her, massaged her, and helped her from her bed to the bedside commode. When she could no longer swallow easily, he prepared baby food for her.

One night he had to telephone Kate and David to come and help him. Magdalena had fallen between the bed and the commode. She weighed ten extra pounds from the swelling and the edema, and Teofilo was too weak from his vigil to get her back into bed.

It was not long after that episode that Magdalena asked Kate why God was making her suffer so much. She wanted Him to take her immediately. Then she fell asleep and Kate tiptoed out of the room. Magdalena awakened an hour later and called for Kate's fifteen-year-old daughter, Mary. Teofilo kept a pistol in a drawer in the next room. Magdalena told Mary to get it. Mary, suspecting nothing, brought it to her grandmother, who said, "Now give it to me." As soon as it was in her hands, she tried to cock it and end her life. Kate said, "It's a good thing the pistol was hard to open and the trigger hard to pull. Of course my father was screaming and I was furious. My daughter was so hurt. Then my mother spoke, very quietly. 'Don't blame Mary. Blame me. It has nothing to do with her.' We were so mad at my mother, but at the same time we knew how she felt and how much she was suffering.

"But that was the only incident like that," Kate said. "So many times in those last months and weeks, my mother would call for Dad, and when he got to her room, she'd just smile at him and say, 'I just wanted to look at you and say I love you.' "

In early October Magdalena began to have moments of irrationality. I explained to the family that it was caused by toxicity from the disease, that it was like being delirious from pneumonia. I also assured them that people usually don't remember what they've said during a toxic phase.

Then one day Teofilo told Kate that her mother refused to take her pills. When Kate urged her to take her medicine, her mother was furious with both of them. After that, she refused to eat, and Kate knew it was time for her mother to go to the hospital. She telephoned her sisters. None of them wanted to suggest such a step to Teofilo. They waited a few days, to let him come to the decision on his own. Kate remembers, "It was a hard thing for him to do. He didn't want to let go of my mother."

I also tried to help Teofilo with his decision, as did Magdalena. I told him a family can do only so much and that there comes a time when special nursing care is needed. Magdalena agreed with the decision, and that helped him too.

During the week that Magdalena spent in the hospital before she died, Teofilo was there all day every day. He went straight to his wife each morning, returned home for lunch at Kate's pleading, and went back to the hospital immediately afterward. Kate or Dely or Victoria would join him there in the afternoons and evenings. Magdalena recognized them only intermittently, and her speech was no longer clear. However, to Kate's relief her mother apologized for speaking to her so angrily the week before. Kate had been worried that her mother would die feeling she had mistreated her.

Speaking of that time, Kate said to me recently, "At first I prayed for a miracle. But after seeing my mother suffer, I hoped it would happen fast. The suffering was too much for her and it was too much for the family.

"Then one day she went into a coma and you told Victoria she might not last the night. We sat by the telephone. It rang at a quarter to one. My father answered it. When he came back into the room he said you had called and my mother had passed away. It was a relief, and yet it was so painful because I knew my Dad would be lost without her. Even when she was in the hospital, at least she was somewhere."

Two days after Magdalena's death, Kate told Dely their father should go to Denver immediately. In two weeks he was home again, but while he was gone Kate and Dely had packed their mother's clothes into a box and stored them in a closet.

"Since that time he's stayed in the room we fixed for him," Kate told me. "But he didn't sell his house. My father is one who keeps things. He's sentimental and he likes to keep good memories.

"At my husband's suggestion Dad took a trip to the Philippines about two months after my mother died. His whole family is there and he hadn't been back in twenty-eight years. While he was there I received a letter from my aunt saying he was quite depressed. They gave him lots of parties and tried to make him happy, but they understood. It was a good trip for him in spite of everything. He took a lot of movies that he now looks at every day."

It is now fifteen months since Magdalena Matunan died. Although Teofilo stays with Kate and her family, he returns to his own home every day. He leaves at midday, visits the cemetery, and spends the remainder of the afternoon in the old house.

Kate says, "At first it broke my heart to see him go there and just sit and watch television. Then one day he said, 'It just makes me feel good to go home.' He feels as though Mom is at work and that she'll be back. I don't know how he feels when it's time for him to leave the house and come back to us. But if that's what makes him happy, nothing else matters.

"My father is a loner. He's at ease with other people, but he doesn't have close friends. He's a family man. He likes to spend his time with his grandchildren, and they're all very fond of him. It makes me happy when I see him smiling and joking around with them, especially my kids and their friends, because they're older and go places with him. He laughs a lot more lately. And he talks much more about my mother. He speaks of her with pride and laughs at some of the things she did.

"Last week he offered rooms in his house to my daughter, who is getting married this spring. It's like seeing myself all over again. I told him they would pay rent, but he got angry and said, 'If your mother were alive, she'd be furious. Are you crazy? Those kids are just getting started.' "

12·When Staff and Fellow Patients Become the Family

For the past nine and a half years I have been associated with a unique hospital that has recently been closed because of administrative changes within the hospital and because the premises did not meet the earthquake requirements of a new state building code. This was the Southern Pacific Railroad Hospital, founded in Sacramento in 1870 and relocated in San Francisco in 1899. The hospital, the first in the world to be built by a railroad for its employees, became a major diagnostic and treatment center for railroad employees. Both young and old employees, retired workers, and many members of their families used the services of the Southern Pacific's prepaid health plan. In 1966 the hospital was renamed the Harkness Community Hospital and Medical Center, and its scope was enlarged to serve private patients from the surrounding community.

The hospital building I worked in was built in 1909, after the 1906 earthquake destroyed the earlier one. Despite its antiquity, the medical facilities, the diagnostic and treatment procedures, and the quality of patient care at Harkness Hospital were excellent. However, its most unusual feature was not its medical excellence but the camaraderie that existed among the patients and between the patients and the hospital staff—nurses and doctors alike. The nurses were devoted to the hospital and some of them had been there for thirty years. The doctors were closely allied and felt little rivalry with each other because they were employed as a group by the hospital association. Among patients who used the medical center frequently many long-lasting friendships were made.

Harkness patients who had cancer usually returned to the hospital every one to three months for a reassessment, staging, and/or therapy. It was the policy of the Oncology Service that any time a patient felt his illness had progressed or that he needed immediate attention, he could admit himself to the hospital. All he had to do was go to Admitting and explain that he was an oncology patient on my service. Thus cancer patients treated at Harkness could feel secure in knowing they would never be denied admission and would receive care whenever they needed it.

The patients were from all over California and often from neighboring states. Those from out of town who came for a diagnostic evaluation or re-evalution were admitted to a boarding ward for three or four days. The nurses and other personnel on the boarding ward were friendly, and the meals were excellent. Family members who came to San Francisco with a patient were helped to find accommodations in the immediate neighborhood.

Patients were usually housed on open wards consisting of twelve to fifteen beds. Private rooms were also available, for a modest additional sum, to those who requested them. On occasion, private rooms were used for patients with communicable infections, and sometimes they were used for patients who were doing poorly, so that families and friends could visit them frequently and stay as long as they wished. Most patients however, seemed to prefer being on the wards. There they and their families exchanged stories about the old days on the railroad and shared their present concerns as well. Patients would call back and forth to each other: "What kind of tumor do you have? What kind of drugs are you taking?" or "Don't get an IV or a bone-marrow from Dr. So-and-so. He's lousy." They were never reticent about grading the performance of their doctors and nurses.

In this friendly, candid atmosphere, the hospital staff, patients, and families became a family for each other. This was especially helpful for patients who had few relatives and friends or who were far from home. Being in the hospital offered a change from a possibly lonely existence. It was a place to go, to be helped, to enjoy the friendly interest of others, and to be regenerated with courage by other patients and the medical staff.

One patient who gave warmth and courage to his fellow patients was Willard Whitmore, a sixty-year-old man with Hodgkin's disease. Willard's cancer was discovered in the spring of 1973, but he had learned to live with cancer in 1949, when his wife became ill with cancer of the intestinal tract. Although she survived a serious operation, she and her husband were told that she did not have long to live. They wondered how soon death would come. This was when Willard decided they must learn to live one day at a time. He recalled, "I told Alice there wasn't any sense worrying about the future because you couldn't tell what it held for anyone. She was very nervous at first. But we made ourselves pay attention to individual days. We walked by the river, got up early to see the sun rise, and sat on the patio to watch the colors change at sunset. Each day there was something special to enjoy."

Twenty-four years later Alice was alive and doing well; Willard was ill. But he announced, "When I told Alice she had to live one day at a time, I learned to do the same thing myself. When you do that, it doesn't make sense to worry about accumulating a lot of money. You don't worry about time or death, either. Everything is destined to live a certain time, like the seasons of the year. When it passes, something new is born. Since that's the way it is, why worry? Besides, worry and fear inhibit your ability to fight disease. As a matter of fact, worry and fear kill more people than disease."

After having his spleen removed, Willard remained in the hospital for a few weeks and then began to commute to San Francisco from his home near Sacramento for radiation therapy. He would stay at the hospital from Monday night until Friday morning, then spend his weekends water-skiing and fishing. Although he had temporary radiation side effects of hair loss and loss of appetite, I never heard him complain. He was gentle and philosophical with everyone, and a sympathetic listener. He wandered through the wards cheering up patients and staff alike. I remember especially a day when he was teasing a friend, Joe, who had just had a lung removed. Joe was terrified and bemoaning his fate when Willard inquired innocently, "Joe, did someone die?"

Joe reminded him that he had lost a lung, whereupon Willard asked, "You mean you don't have a lung left?"

"No," Joe explained further. "They took one lung. I still have the other."

Willard winked and looked perplexed, "Well, what are you complaining for? The time to worry is when you lose the other one."

Willard gave each patient the benefit of his wisdom, on subjects from acupuncture to water-skiing, from being able to discern which doctor gave painless injections to the advantages of living in the country.

Occasionally there was a patient whom not even Willard could reach. Roger Cook was such a person. For him the hospital was just a place to go. In addition to being a retired railroad employee, he was a veteran of World War II and therefore had a second option of going to a veterans' hospital. We know little else of Roger's past beyond a few facts on his medical record and a short acquaintance with him in the hospital. Born in 1912, he told us he had lived alone since being discharged from the army in 1945. In 1943 he had gotten a divorce after a brief marriage. He then became a ticket seller for the Southern Pacific Railroad and remained in that job for twenty years, retiring in 1968 in Los Angeles.

Roger seemed to have minimal contact with two surviving sisters, but apparently he had been close to a brother who died in early July 1971. A week after his brother's death, Roger was admitted to Harkness for the first time, suffering from depression and severe headaches. Two months later, in September, he was readmitted for the same reason. Although Roger denied feeling depressed and having thoughts of suicide, he did admit that he often stayed in bed most of the day, going to bed at midnight and arising around eleven in the morning, sometimes not bothering to get up until late afternoon. A report by the psychiatric consultant stated that Roger was depressed and that his depression was being manifested through physical symptoms.

Two years later, in June 1973, Roger returned to Harkness for a re-evaluation in the Medical Service. He said he had lost thirty pounds in six months. On physical examination a mass was found in his right flank, and an exploratory laparotomy revealed a large mass in his right kidney, with superficial invasion of the liver. Roger was subsequently seen by the doctors in the Oncology Service, where we explained his diagnosis to him and began treatment with hormone injections. He either did not understand or refused to acknowledge his problem and the desirability of continuing hormonal therapy, and did not follow our recommendations for continuing treatment when he returned to Los Angeles. We did not see him again until three months later, when he asked to be readmitted to Harkness. By then he had lost an additional ten pounds and complained that his right leg was swollen and tender.

When I arrived on the ward the morning following Roger's readmittance, he was lying on his side, awake. His body was bent and worn, his thin face covered with a stubble of gray. He was frightened and in pain. We talked for a little while. I asked him whether he knew what was wrong with him, but he didn't want to say. I told him he had a tumor, but his only response was, "You fix up my leg and I'll be all right." Such a comment is not unusual. A patient will often be more concerned about what is hurting at the moment than about his major medical problem, which in Roger's case was metastatic cancer. I told Roger we would treat his leg and that we could help relieve his pain, but I also tried to convey to him the gravity of his disease. He began to cry. He then asked to be transferred to a veterans' hospital in Southern California, near one of his sisters, though he admitted that he had not seen or corresponded with her in years.

We began to make the necessary arrangements for Roger's transfer. In the meantime he rarely spoke to anyone, although he never took his eyes off the doctors as we made our rounds and talked with other patients. He never asked questions except to inquire in a belligerent manner, "When will my leg get better?" He also watched very closely a patient across the room whose family visited frequently. This family and other people, including the house staff and the nurses, would try to talk to Roger. He seemed terrified of being alone and of dying, yet he was unable to respond to their many gestures of friendship. He continued to cry intermittently. He was in pain but he refused medication, saying there was no point in taking it.

We explained and offered to Roger the available cancer therapies and assured him that we would do everything possible to make him comfortable if he would give us his cooperation. He was furious that we could offer him so little and convinced that he would receive more effective treatment at the veterans' hospital. But before we could complete the arrangements for his transfer, he announced one morning, "What's the use," packed his belongings, and, barely able to walk, departed for Los Angeles. Before he left, we told him there would always be a bed for him at Harkness if he wasn't satisfied with the veterans' hospital. We never heard from him again. A follow-up phone call to his sister revealed that Roger had died in the veterans' hospital a month after he left us.

It was Roger's choice to live by himself. However, when he became ill, he needed help, and after the death of his brother there appeared to be no one with whom he could share his problems. When he was finally offered support and friendship at Harkness, he was unable to accept them. That he could not talk about his sadness and his fears was a sorrow to those of us who tried to reach him. He seemed not to have the capacity to participate in the unique system of group therapy and mutual help that had evolved at Harkness.

13 · The Cancer Patient Who Lives Alone

When their condition permits it, many patients prefer to receive treatment as outpatients, so that they can remain at home. This is not difficult when home consists of adequate living facilities and friends or family members who can help out when needed. Unfortunately, not every patient has such ideal circumstances at home, and it is not easy for a doctor to know which of his patients may need more help than he is getting. This was my experience with Arthur English.

Once a robust man, Arthur, at sixty-two, had metastatic colon cancer with bladder involvement. He had a colostomy on his abdomen and a urinary catheter attached to a bag on his thigh. He had been referred to me a year after his surgery, and in the year and a half since then I had found him cheerful and outgoing, despite his cancer problems. Talking with him was always a pleasant experience.

Although Arthur lived alone in a hotel near the financial district in San Francisco, I never thought of him as a lonely man. He had many concerned friends who would phone me frequently to find out what could be done to help him. Arthur was from Oklahoma and still had close relatives there, but he frankly admitted that they irritated him after a short time, so he limited contact with them to occasional brief visits.

While Arthur was under my care, he always preferred to be treated as an outpatient for his therapy and his blood transfusions. He said he had been hospitalized too often in the past. However, on one of his visits to my office for therapy, I found that Arthur was very run-down— anemic, exhausted, and unable to eat satisfactorily. As these symptoms increased, he was less able to tolerate chemotherapy, and I suggested that he be hospitalized so we could rebuild his strength. Arthur said he would think it over, and we made an appointment for him to come to my office again the following week.

When Arthur failed to keep the appointment, I phoned him. He said he needed some rest and would come the next week. Once again he failed to appear. This time Isadora phoned him and reported to me that Arthur sounded sad and depressed. She also said he hesitated and did not give a clear answer when she asked whether he would like me to make a house call. He muttered something about being fine. That evening I decided to visit Arthur to make sure he was all right.

I had known that Arthur lived in a somewhat shabby residential hotel, but I was unprepared for some of the physical hardships he had to endure in addition to his cancer. He lived in one room which contained a bed, two dressers, two wooden chairs, and a wash basin. A blender, a coffee maker, some packets of instant breakfast, and other items were crowded onto a table next to a hot plate. On the hot plate was a frying pan with a small amount of dried-up food. A clean quilt was thrown across the bed where Arthur lay, and his favorite books and cherished possessions were on top of the dresser and stacked around the room.

These accommodations would have been bearable if they had not lacked a private bathroom. At best it must have been difficult and distressing for Arthur to perform colostomy irrigations in the shared bathroom at the end of the hall.

Arthur explained that he had not been back for chemotherapy because he had been weakened by a severe attack of diarrhea after his therapy two weeks earlier. He hadn't mentioned his condition to me on the telephone. Even now he wasn't complaining; he was merely telling me in a matter-of-fact voice what the trouble was. He then apologized because his room was in a state of disarray and had not been cleaned while he was sick. I had been acquainted with Arthur long enough to know he was an orderly, fastidious person, immaculate in dress and in the care of his colostomy. He was a man of great dignity, proud of his self-sufficiency, and was now embarrassed to have me see how he was living.

After I examined him we talked again about the possibility of his being hospitalized, and he agreed to let me send for him in a few days. The reason for the delay was that he wanted to put his room in order. I then realized that Arthur had no telephone either, and that whenever we called him he had to walk to the hall phone and talk standing up. A few days later, according to our agreement, I arranged hospitalization and sent an ambulance for him.

There are many people who live alone and who, like Arthur, are either too proud to accept help or simply don't want it, even though their illness has incapacitated them and brought upheaval and disorganization to their lives. Doctors may not realize how often this situation occurs, or what other essentials of home care may be lacking. I did not realize until I visited him what Arthur went through when he had diarrhea and had to care for his colostomy several times in one day. I also did not realize that he could have used help with cleaning and cooking from time to time. I am certain Arthur's friends would have been glad to help him, but Arthur, like many other people, did not want to ask. I can understand such reticence and admire the obvious courage it implies, but that attitude is not realistic. If the patient who prefers not to ask his family or friends for favors will at least be candid with his doctor about his needs, the doctor may direct him to one of the social service agencies whose function is to provide assistance in such matters. Their help can make a substantial difference in the basic every-day comfort and convenience that are needed to make living with cancer a little more tolerable.

Part V
The Will to Live

14 · Anthony Verdi

"I had a total conviction that I would be all right. I never once considered myself a leukemia victim. I never bought your philosophy, Rosie. You said I had to respect the disease, but I said, 'No way. I don't respect it at all because the moment I do, I'll be afraid of it, and fear is the greatest enemy in this thing.'"

"But you acknowledge that you had leukemia," I reminded Anthony.

"Yes. I had the disease. I created it and I got rid of it."

"How does chemotherapy fit into your philosophy?" I continued.

"Chemotherapy was a crutch, and I was willing to go along with all the crutches. I was willing to use any means available until I was able to do it myself."

"You know I don't agree with your theories, Anthony, but I won't fight them either. It will be many years before research will supply us with answers to some of the issues you raise. Whichever of us is right, one of my rules is 'Don't knock success.' Some people would agree with you, however, and others would be interested in what you have to say. Would you describe your experience with leukemia—your medical treatment, and your own views on the cause and control of disease?"

"I'd be glad to."

The symptoms came upon me gradually, just after I turned twenty-six. In March 1970, about six months before my diagnosis, I began to feel tired more easily than usual. By summer my fatigue was even more pronounced. I was bleeding from the gums, but I reasoned that that was because of a baby tooth that had never been replaced.

The discovery of my condition was even postponed by a couple of coincidences. In August I had to go to an army summer camp and I was supposed to have a blood test the day before I left, but I didn't know that I was supposed to fast before a blood test, so they didn't give it to me. I spent two weeks in the camp and felt pretty good although I was still somewhat tired. The only other unusual physical symptoms were blood blisters on my feet that failed to heal.

The blood test that I missed was rescheduled for September 12, after my return, but I had to cancel the appointment because I was an usher at a wedding. I didn't have the test until the next Saturday. That day I noticed the first hematoma on my right arm. By the next night I had four or five hematomas on other parts of my body. Monday morning I consulted my internist, who referred me to you.

During the previous week I had taken a leave of absence from my job to attend law school full time. However, I noticed that I was taking three or four times longer than usual to make decisions or to function in any way. To check out all these symptoms I looked through a layman's handbook on medicine the night before I saw my internist, so I already guessed that I might have a blood disease of some sort. I just didn't know which one.

I entered the hospital for tests on Tuesday, September 21. Blood and bone-marrow tests were performed. When the diagnosis was confirmed, you and your Fellow took me into the nurses' room. You both looked grave. You told me I had acute leukemia.

I experienced a momentary panic, during which I thought, "Why me?" That didn't last more than a second or two because at the same moment I decided I was going to lick it. The reason for the quickness of my decision and the stabilization of my emotions is that I had been practicing a way of thinking, a way of life, for many years. This philosophy has an approach toward cancer, as well as other diseases, that is based on the belief that every disease, although real, is psychosomatically induced. There are no exceptions. The emotional and mental state of the individual triggers the germs and viruses in the body that create disease. I therefore knew I was responsible for creating the climate that allowed leukemia to develop and that I was just as responsible for changing that climate in order to conquer it. I also subscribe to the notion that anything can be done if you believe in it strongly enough, and this includes the eradication of disease. You can even kid yourself about what you believe as long as you realize you're kidding yourself—just so there's no internal conflict. There are no defeats, only wins. Even the defeats have an element of win in them. You have to concentrate all your attention on that one little element of win and drop the rest.

I knew why I was vulnerable to leukemia. My marriage had recently broken up and I was very depressed. I was depressed because the relationship was destroyed, not because I was particularly in love with my ex-wife at that point. I was also having problems at work. The people there were bugging me. I had been given extra jobs to do, and I was being criticized for not being able to do them as they wanted me to. Therefore there was a series of resentments and rejections that had a lot to do with my emotional state.

Another thing that calmed me down when you gave me my diagnosis was that I said to myself, "I don't care whether I live or die." This also helped eliminate volcanic emotional eruptions because I then went on to think, "Okay, but there are some worthwhile things to live for." Then I began ticking them off. "This would be nice and that would be nice." Going through this process cleared me of panic, and I was able to think calmly, "Let's hear them out." The technical term for my acute leukemia was promyelocytic. I was told I had two alternatives. I could do nothing, or I could take chemotherapy. I decided on the latter, which was what you recommended. I was also to receive blood transfusions.

You told me a little about chemotherapy, how the drugs were strong but that they were no longer experimental. We decided to begin the next day with a five-day course of multidrug chemotherapy. I had never had my veins punctured in any way, except for an occasional blood test, and that became a traumatic new experience, because it was done more than once or twice a day. However, you and the Fellow had told me about the advantages of giving chemotherapy by IV. You also tried to reduce the number of blood tests per day, and you drew the blood and serviced the IVs yourselves in order to save my veins.

I was never afraid while receiving chemotherapy, but as the drugs entered my body, there was a cold feeling. It wasn't necessarily clammy or distasteful, just a cold feeling that lasted anywhere from a few minutes to half an hour. Although I felt subjectively that my temperature had been lowered, I know that wasn't the case.

At that time my blood counts were extremely low; I had about 300 to 500 white blood cells, as opposed to a normal count of over 5,000. I had no platelets, and I had many immature, or blastic, leukemia cells. You also told me I was to receive an anticoagulant because with my particular form of leukemia there was clotting in my blood vessels. I was also bleeding internally, and I was tired.

The five-day course of chemotherapy was followed by a ten-day rest, and then the cycle would be repeated. The objective during that initial phase of treatment was to destroy the malignant cells in the bone marrow. Of course, the longer I was on chemotherapy, the weaker I got. During the ten days that I was off the drugs, I often had a fever.

You were a tremendous boost to me at that time. You were cheerful in front of me and conveyed great hope, although privately I think you felt I was a lost cause because you had seen so many similar cases. I didn't pick up any negative thinking, however; I was too busy trying to convince you and my parents that everything would be all right. You showed your faith and optimism when you phoned the law school and asked for a leave of absence for me and arranged that I could go back the following year.

As I look back, I believe my basic determination to get well never left me. Not once. During the first three or four weeks, when I wasn't completely wiped out, I was very cheerful, bantering with you and the nurses, and trying to cheer up my parents and friends. Then the fevers began to get worse. In fact, during October and November I had fevers of 104 and 105 degrees daily for a three-week period and was in a semicomatose state. You controlled my fever with an ice blanket, ice packs, and antibiotics and other medicines. I became delirious and also had a mild stroke. I had extremely heavy headaches which you thought might be due to a small brain hemorrhage. And I lost my hair bit by bit. I was put in reverse isolation several times so I wouldn't pick up infections.

One of the funniest things was that when I had my stroke I was convinced I was all right and hadn't had a stroke. A neurologist came in and examined me, and even though I was wiped out, with no bone marrow, I performed feats like jumping on one foot and running up and down the hall, through sheer will power, to prove to him that I was all right. Brain scans, EEGs, and other tests were made, but the exact cause of the stroke was never determined. You said it could have been from bleeding because of the low platelet count or from the toxic effect of the drugs.

During that three-week period of high fever and delirium a friend came to visit me who shares the same ideas I do. He looked at me and said, "Gee, Anthony, that's a marvelous game you're playing." That's all he said. The next day my fever came down to 99, and from then on I was fairly stable.

That autumn of 1970 I was in the hospital for three months, from September 21 to the end of December. During that time I received one hundred and five units of blood. They consisted of platelets for bleeding and red blood cells for anemia. When my leukemia was announced where my dad works, and at law school, which I'd only attended for a week, there was a spontaneous offering of blood donations. The blood transfusions produced a rushing feeling. It must be like the rushing feeling people speak of who are on amphetamines or STP. It was a very uncomfortable sensation, as though things were rushing through me. I later had hepatitis, probably from the blood, because my serum liver function tests were abnormal.

Within that three-month time span I did sink into moods similar to depression, but they were mainly apathy. My thoughts were always positive, though. I knew—I didn't just hope—that everything would be okay. I remember telling you that in January 1971. You said, "Why didn't you tell me in September?" and I replied, "You wouldn't have believed me."

While I was in the hospital my parents were there morning, noon, and night. Dad and mother would both take time off from work. They were completely devoted parents. After I had been there two months I could no longer eat the food, either for taste or for psychological reasons. My mouth was full of sores and I could only eat pureed food. So Ma would fix pureed food for me. I am from Argentina and we have a Spanish–Latin American tradition of very close family ties, so although such acts of devotion aren't necessarily expected, they just seem like the natural things that parents do for children. No sacrifice is too great for any member of the family. So to me it was not an unusual thing for my mother to do that, although everyone was commenting on it, saying, "You're being spoiled. You're depending too much on your parents. It's an unnatural relationship."

One thing that helped me a lot during those months was the number of people with whom I became involved. It was fascinating, because people that I'd never met before, total strangers, would come in and want to talk to me. Of course I always went out of my way to make them feel comfortable and welcomed in my room. I was also extremely touched and flattered by their warmth and friendship because I knew they really cared for me. One of my favorites was a nurse from England, a brilliant guy named Fleur Stanley, who did a great deal for my morale. He was a no-nonsense individual and very witty. He was a positive person with lots of determination. He had a psychological plan for me. He visited me at a certain time each day, and we would have a fifteen-minute talk on some subject of interest. We'd discuss these ideas back and forth, and of course he'd never believe anything I'd say, and I'd tease him.

Once or twice I had a problem with the other nurses, however, because they would get too emotionally involved with me. I think this tends to happen especially when a patient is young and seriously ill. There was one particular student nurse who spent too much time in my room. I was asked whether she was bothering me and if I wanted her transferred, but I said, "No. She can stay." She was transferred to another floor anyway. I had told her myself many times, "Look, you've been here long enough. You'd better go do your other duties." I think this kind of problem arose because I didn't give a damn about what anybody thought of my ideas, and I seem to be a person that people like to tell their problems to. In turn, I would give them the benefit of my philosophy and tell them what they could do if they wanted to. This young nurse listened to me, was impressed by what I said, and apparently became infatuated.

At the end of December 1970 I was shocked to find out that I was in remission, because that meant that I had to leave the hospital. The hospital had become my home and I didn't want to leave. I was happy that the remission had come about as I had wanted it to, but going home was less exciting than being in the hospital, where people are more apt to visit you. I wanted that attention, and I think that feeling fostered the problem I sometimes had with the nurses. Anyway, I had formed a lot of fast friendships in the hospital, and I didn't want to lose the daily contact. The support of these friends meant love, that people really cared about me. And that was another factor in what I believe induced my illness. I had wanted everybody to love me. I no longer feel this way. Before, if anyone showed any kind of ill will or reaction against me, I instantly thought he or she hated me or didn't like me, and this would totally depress me. I didn't spend my time peering around every corner to see if people liked me, but there were certain times when I felt that way.

Those reactions have been diminishing for years, as I have learned to handle such feelings on my own. It was part of a pattern of thinking in which I felt that at some point the environment was at fault for things that happened to me. In other words, *they* did it to me. I now believe the opposite is true, that anything that happens to me I have caused in some way, even if it is a razor-thin responsibility on my part. My share of the responsibility may only be the fact that I was there to receive the stimulus from the outside. I am responsible for being there, for receiving it, and finally for how I react to it. With anything that has a cause outside myself —even if it's someone menacing me, or acting as if he hates my guts—it is still within my power to react one way or the other and in that way to exert control over my own life. That is to say, I can believe the game that guy out there is playing and respond with either "How terrible. He hates me" or "What the hell is bothering him so much that he has to feel that way about me?"

At home during the month of January 1971 I spent most of my time on my back because I was very weak. I had gone from 192 pounds down to 150 since September. The disease and the drugs had weakened me so that running across the street was enough to make my knees collapse. In fact I fell down one time. But even though I was weak, I was in partial remission and I felt clean and purged inside.

Between January 1971 and June 1971 I went to the hospital for one week each month for chemotherapy and would be off for three weeks. In May I came down with a fever and an infection. I don't know what caused it, but I was admitted to the hospital for four days in reverse isolation. My white blood cells were down to 500 again, and I was given a blood transfusion and antibiotic therapy for the infection. It lasted approximately seven days, but this time when I left the hospital I no longer felt I was leaving a nice place. In five months I had adjusted to being out of the hospital and had no desire to return.

My total remission came sometime during that year, 1971. I re-enrolled in law school in September and was put on maintenance therapy, a reduced chemotherapeutic program. I would spend three days in the hospital every four weeks, to receive the intravenous part of the therapy, and would complete the cycle by taking tablets at home.

I continued in this way until January 30, 1972, when I had a coronary and had to spend eighteen days in the hospital. My cardiologist, Dr. Gordon Katznelson, felt that the tension of going back to law school would aggravate my heart problem, so he phoned the school and arranged for another leave of absence. I can understand his reasoning, but if he hadn't done that, I would probably have faked it and gone back and finished with no problems. He didn't understand the way I felt about things. I never explained my philosophy to him.

From that time until I returned to law school the next September I kept myself busy seeing friends and doing all kinds of things. I took the real estate license exam and I went to Argentina for thirty-five days.

I continued with a maintenance dose of chemotherapy, but on a schedule that allowed me more independence than before. Then, Rosie, you would insert a small IV tube in my vein that would remain for several days, and I could go home and inject the chemotherapy into the tubing myself. I also continued with the chemotherapy tablets. You would see me once a day for five days each month, to check my blood and supply the drugs for the next injection. This program of chemotherapy lasted until August 1973, when I decided I didn't want any more. You discussed the possibility of immunotherapy or brain radiation, but I had a negative reaction to both suggestions. I don't know how much you were aware of my feelings. I hope I was diplomatic, but I felt I didn't need any more therapy. I felt fine.

Therefore, in August I went off chemotherapy of all kinds. I also stopped taking the oral antibiotic that I had been on for three years to guard against skin infection. It is now May 1975, and I've been off chemotherapy for twenty months. I'm feeling marvelous. I remember when I quit, I said to myself, "At last you had the courage to go off that stuff."

"Anthony, that was an accurate account of the last three and a half years, but you forgot to mention that you got married six months ago to one of my favorite nurses, that you have graduated from law school and taken the bar examination. But back to your decision to stop therapy. I did not agree with that decision, but I also did not have an exact answer on how much longer we should continue some form of therapy. You were in a fortunate state to stop treatment when you did, and it worked. Since August 1973 we've watched you closely. At first we performed bone-marrow tests every three weeks, then at six-week intervals; and now we only do a test every two months. We're relying on your body to take over and defend itself, but if there is ever a recurrence of your leukemia we'll treat it as we did before. How would you feel if you had a recurrence, Anthony?"

"No problem," was his prompt reply. "If I got a recurrence, I'd know I created it. If I'm willing to play that game again, then what the hell am I doing, that's all. But I certainly would not panic."

"You say you didn't respect your disease, but when we explained to you how we wanted to treat it, you were cooperative, and that was important," I said. "You and I have been talking about the desire to live that is in all of us. Our philosophies about how to accomplish a cure are different, but we both know the will to live makes a difference, and that patients who have this desire to survive fight harder and do better medically than those who lack the drive. It's an intangible, unmeasurable force that makes a difference."

"I believe it makes all the difference," Anthony replied. "If you have the faith that you're going to make it, if you have the will to win, you'll make it. And if you introduce any doubts, you've had it."

I nodded. "But many people *say* they're going to beat their disease."

"The difference is, they don't believe it. In the back of their minds they're saying, "You fool. You're really kidding yourself.""

"Are you being completely fair about that?" I asked. "The will to live is important, and if a person is convinced he will get well, that's even better. But we know of no specific effect on cancer cells that is caused by a positive state of mind."

"I know you don't agree with some of my ideas," Anthony said patiently, "but I know that even when I kid myself into feeling something, once I acquire the feeling, it's a true feeling. It's the feeling you're going to be okay. You convince yourself. You know you have something, and you say, 'Well, I'm going to have something else instead, something that's healthy. What would it be like to feel healthy right now, even though I'm sick?' In that way you begin to create a future for yourself. When you do that, you're not thinking about how you have this dread disease that will kill you. You shift your focus, your concentration, away from the disease, even though you are still aware of it.

"That's just my understanding of health in me," Anthony added. "It might not apply to someone else's way of thinking. I was totally convinced. It's that simple. I knew, just as I know that the sun is going to rise tomorrow, even if I don't see it—I knew that I would be healthy again."

Part VI
Supportive Services

15 · Nurses

The nurse plays a key role in patient care. During a patient's stay in the hospital, 80 percent of his contact with hospital personnel is under the guidance and direction of the nursing staff. If he has cancer, he may be tended by an oncology nurse who has received special training in the care and treatment of cancer patients. In some hospitals there are now special units for cancer care similar to the coronary unit for heart disease.

I interviewed three nurses* who work exclusively with cancer patients. I was particularly interested in finding out how they felt about cancer nursing after several years of experience, and how they dealt with their own emotional responses, as well as those of the patients and their families.

ER: Why did you go into cancer nursing?

EILEEN SHEPLEY: I think it's one of the more satisfying kinds of nursing. The patients are fantastic to work with, despite their anxieties and fears. In comparison with the average internal medical patient, cancer patients have fewer pretenses. They readily accept the side effects of therapy because of their will to live, and they are more responsive to the support and encouragement of doctors and nurses. Another reason I like cancer nursing is the feeling I have of being needed.

MARY LAWTON: I came to cancer nursing in a roundabout way. My prior nursing experience had been one of defeat, and I thought it was something I never wanted to encounter again. I was de-

* Mary Lawton, R.N., oncology nurse, formerly at Mount Zion Hospital and Medical Center, San Francisco; Eileen Shepley, R.N., oncology nurse, Claire Zellerbach Saroni Tumor Institute, Mount Zion Hospital and Medical Center; and Fleur Frederick Stanley, S.R.N., O.N.C., West Middlesex Hospital, London, England, Nursing Administrative Supervisor, Mount Zion Hospital and Medical Center, San Francisco.

pressed. I had found it difficult and painful to work with patients who were ill, undergoing therapy, or dying. Then, because of a series of circumstances, I found I needed a job, and Memorial Hospital in New York City was the only place with an opening. I thought, "Necessity has brought me to something I'm not going to be able to handle." Instead, I found I was very comfortable at Memorial Hospital and liked it enormously. I'm not sure why. Perhaps I had reached a level of personal development that made it possible for me to relax and face all the problems that had once seemed so overwhelming. Also, I began to realize that cancer nursing was the most rewarding kind. Before I went to Memorial Hospital I was bored with nursing. In contrast, although emotionally taxing, cancer nursing is challenging and gratifying.

You can do so much for cancer patients that doctors don't have time to do by offering them something personal. To follow through after receiving a doctor's orders isn't enough. There are many situations in which a doctor may say, "You take care of it. You know more than I do." For example, when a patient has a colostomy, a nurse can teach him how to take care of it. A colostomy can be a traumatic experience for a patient. The help he receives from the nurse is real and useful.

ER: Mrs. Shepley, what qualities and skills do you think are most essential in a good cancer nurse?

ES: I think she has to have a genuine concern for other people to be a good nurse, but especially to be a good cancer nurse. She has to be willing to become involved and give of herself, even though it means she will be hurt when patients suffer a relapse or die. She also needs a good theoretical and practical background in communication and interpersonal relationships. This helps her in supporting the patient and his family. The important thing is to be able to sit down and talk with a patient and to reassure him that someone cares.

A good cancer nurse also has to have a broad background of knowledge and skill. She needs experience in specific procedures such as colostomy and tracheotomy care. She must be skilled in doing procedures because cancer patients are very good at detecting indecision and lack of skill. They often equate getting well with how efficiently a procedure is carried out, whether it involves an IV, chemotherapy, or another kind of therapy. If a nurse is not adept, a patient may think his chances of recovery are reduced.

ER: How do your patients respond to you?

ES: At first most patients are fearful and anxious, but after we've worked together for a while they become more relaxed. A large part of a nurse's job is to help alleviate anxiety. Hers is a supportive, sharing role. She must be able to interpret and integrate a patient's problems into the plan of medical therapy and acknowledge the feasibility of what can be done for him.

ER: Mr. Stanley, you're a nursing supervisor on a floor where the majority are cancer patients. Would you describe a typical day and some of the problems that may arise?

FLEUR STANLEY: When I come onto the floor each day, I look through the patients' files and I see what changes have occurred and what notes have been made. I also talk with the nurses who are going off duty to find out if there are any new problems from the day before. When I have analyzed the data, I have a good sense of what I want to do and set up the plan for that day.

Often a nurse will tell me that a patient has asked me to drop by his room if I am "not too busy." Then I know that the patient has something on his mind that he wishes to discuss with me. This kind of visit is of critical importance. The patient needs an opportunity to voice his pent-up feelings. He needs a person who will encourage him to blow off steam without taking what he says too personally and becoming defensive. A nurse should know that a patient who is irritable or irate is rarely angry at her. More likely, he is angry with someone else—a relative, perhaps—or at his illness, but is unable to admit his frustration. He has to do something with his anger, so he directs it at whoever is around. If the nurse can accept the bitterness and the anger and talk with the patient about it, she may enable him to explore what's really on his mind.

Other tense situations may occur. The person with cancer is often apprehensive. Any treatment he is receiving is a major issue because he feels his life depends on it. When he puts on the light that summons the nurse, it must be answered immediately. For example, if a patient is on intravenous therapy and the IV should become empty and need replacement, the patient will turn on the light and call the nurse. "The IV is out! You know that's important to me. I need it. You shouldn't have allowed it to happen." He's really saying, "Look what I'm going through!"

The daily menu provides another object for the ventilation of frustration and apprehension. A patient may become extra sensitive regarding any item of food that doesn't come up to his expectations. That everything be properly done is essential because he must get well. Each slight inconvenience becomes a major event over which he can express his constant fear of being neglected.

ER: But the patient isn't the only one who presents problems.

FS: Certainly not. In some cases the nurse can be the cause of a problem. One afternoon I went into a patient's room and sensed immediately that something was wrong between the patient and his special duty nurse. Afterward, I took another nurse aside and told her to ask the patient, when she was next alone in his room, what was wrong. It turned out that the patient's morning nurse completed her duty at three o'clock but that the afternoon nurse was always forty-five minutes late. The morning nurse resented having to stay until her replacement arrived. Animosity had built up between them and it was making the patient uncomfortable. Naturally, he was reluctant to speak about it in front of the nurse who was causing the trouble. Asking him while she was out of the room enabled us to find out quickly what was wrong and to replace her.

ER: When a patient is admitted to the hospital, the staff's first concern is whether he has been informed of his diagnosis, or, if he has been informed, whether he has accepted it. Occasionally, too, as you have all experienced, a patient may not have been given an adequate explanation of his illness. In such a situation, a patient is puzzled or fearful and may ask the nurse if she knows the answer to his medical problem or the meaning of his diagnosis. Even when a patient has been told his diagnosis, he may ask the nurse for confirmation and explanation. She, of course, cannot give that explanation without first obtaining the permission of the patient's physician. What has been your experience with uninformed, or inadequately informed, patients?

FS: Very often a patient who is not adequately informed about his condition has a doctor who doesn't want to become emotionally involved with him or his family. You can tell which doctors are like this by watching them with a patient. They will practically run into the room, have a quick chat, and depart as soon as possible to avoid a direct confrontation with the patient. I have often observed this pattern of behavior and sometimes try to help the patient by telephoning the doctor and asking him, "Did you explain the problem to the family? Does the patient want to know his diagnosis?"

ML: Most patients, of course, are told their diagnoses, but doctors vary as to how well they explain it or how frank they are with a patient. I think most nurses are disappointed with doctors who are not sufficiently candid. A lot of doctors feel that once they have told a patient he has cancer, there is no need for further discussion. For most people this is a shattering experience. They need to have the details repeated several times before they can begin to comprehend and accept their situation. I think the reason some doctors don't want to talk about the diagnosis in detail is simply that it makes them feel helpless and therefore uncomfortable. They just don't want to communicate bad news to a patient.

A doctor's reluctance to talk openly can initiate a cycle of isolation and noncommunication. A triangle develops, with the patient thinking his thoughts, the nurse her thoughts, and the doctor his thoughts. This can cause resentment in the patient, who is, after all, the person who matters most. He probably knows what he has and how bad it is, but there is no one with whom he can talk. Thus, in addition to suffering through denial and depression, he will also feel alienated from the health professionals who should be building his trust and confidence.

A lack of communication can also interfere with treatment. A patient who has not sufficiently understood his medical problems and prospects may be reluctant or afraid to undergo therapy.

FS: It's not always a matter of whether a patient knows his diagnosis or of how well it's been presented to him, but of whether he wants to know it and has accepted it. Usually, if you listen very carefully, the answer is apparent. Sometimes a patient will refer to his "symptoms," his "complaint," or his "illness." Eventually he may enlarge on that and say, "I think it's a tumor." He may even refer to his malignancy as "cancer." When he reaches this stage, you realize he not only knows but accepts his diagnosis.

However, there are some patients who will tell you outright, "I don't want to know. Don't tell me." If that's what a patient wants, it's perfectly all right, although even this patient inwardly knows the truth. If you watch him carefully, you'll see his knowledge manifested in depression, anger, frustration, or a need for attention. Comments such as "The food's not good enough," "It's too hot," "It's too cold," "It doesn't taste right," or "I can't sleep. My bed's uncomfortable" reveal his state of mind. Once you actually sit down and talk to such a patient and help him understand his diagnosis, his behavior may change.

ER: Mrs. Shepley, how do you reduce anxiety in a patient and/or help him accept his diagnosis?

ES: It isn't so much what I do as how I interact with a patient that reduces his anxiety. I can communicate my warmth and interest simply by being with him. I follow no rules. Sometimes I find a point of common interest. It may be family life, children, sports, travel, or whatever. As we become better acquainted with each other, it becomes easier for him to talk. It's also important that I be relaxed. If I can convey a degree of calm and serenity, a patient who is uptight may relax and begin to express his feelings. I may touch a shoulder or pat an arm. It depends on the patient but almost all of them like a feeling of closeness. As I said before, a patient associates the cancer nurse, as well as his doctor, with his hope for recovery.

ER: A patient who has difficulty confiding in his doctor may have more courage to speak to his nurse. A sensitive nurse will be alert to such a dilemma and consult the attending physician as to how they can best handle the situation.

At other times a patient may never have had the opportunity during his doctor's routine visits to ask him all the questions that bother him. Again, the nurse can be an effective intermediary between patient and doctor. Mr. Stanley, how do you go about finding out what's really troubling a patient?

FS: I find it best not to ask direct questions. When a patient appears upset, there's a tendency to ask him "What's the matter?" or "What's bothering you?" The form of the question suggests that there's something wrong with the patient or that he's behaving badly. Patients suffer enough indignities without receiving additional insults. I find that an indirect statement that doesn't require an answer is most effective in encouraging a patient to share his feelings. "You seem to be upset about something" or "I can tell there's something on your mind" indicates to a patient that I'm aware of how he feels and offer him a choice as to whether he will share his thoughts at that time.

ER: Such a patient may be afraid, among other things. In what ways do you detect fear, and how do you help a patient who is afraid?

FS: One of the most common feelings a patient conceals is fear. Although some people will be quite frank and tell you, "I'm scared stiff," most people don't like to admit they're afraid; and many are afraid without knowing it. Concealed fear may be expressed as depression, withdrawal, or a need for diversion. The most common reaction to fear is withdrawal, where a patient just sleeps for long periods of time. Diversion includes any ordinary behavior carried to an extreme. Some patients read voraciously, day and night; others play their television or radio at high volume for hours; and some joke continuously and refuse to talk about anything serious. These same people are subject to the complaints, outbursts of temper, and other signs of emotional strain that I mentioned. When we have such a patient on the floor, I take time to go into his room, sit down, and talk with him. At some point in the conversation I ask him if he is frightened, and why. He may deny his feelings, but more often he will admit he is afraid. I may then tell him I think I would feel as he does.

I do the same thing with the family. I may see the wife of a patient crying. She will apologize, saying she can't help it, and I will tell her, "This is a normal reaction. You don't like to see your husband this way. You're hurt." It usually works. The wife is relieved of the pressure of having to control her feelings, and she is less reluctant to talk about them.

ER: Miss Lawton, how do you relate to the families of patients?

ML: This depends in part on how the members of a family interpret the nurse's role. Some people see the nurse as an authority figure, while others see her simply as a worker. When the doctor isn't available, one family may be content with talking to the nurse. Another family may say "No" very emphatically when I ask whether I can be of help. Still other families never even ask to speak to the doctor but seek all their information from the nurse.

ER: Mr. Stanley, what do you see as the advantages and disadvantages of a family's presence and participation in the hospital care of a patient?

FS: Relatives are frequently in a highly anxious state and may have a pronounced effect on the patient. It's not unusual for them to spend enormous amounts of time with him, to the extent of sleeping in his room. Often they feel responsibility or guilt for the patient's illness and try to assuage it with overattentiveness. This diligence may express itself through impatience with the hospital services, or through a sense of urgency similar to the apprehensiveness expressed by the patient himself.

The mother of a young boy with Hodgkin's disease practically lived in her son's room and was constantly critical of the nursing care he was receiving. Once she asked me to get her son a mouthwash, and when I did not reappear with it instantly, she ran into the hall, grabbed my coat, and shook me, screaming that I was ignoring her child's needs. I took the woman's arms, held her firmly, and said, "Calm down. I'm going to get the mouthwash in a few minutes. Now, please sit here in the nursing station and drink a cup of coffee." I wanted to reassert a sense of priorities so she would realize that a mouthwash was not an acute medical necessity.

An inexperienced nurse may tend to view relatives as impediments and try to work around them. She will acknowledge their presence and try to accommodate them without compromising her duties. However, she will soon learn that a family's participation in the care of a patient can be advantageous to herself, the patient, and his family. The family's ability to do things for the patient frees her for other duties, gives the patient a sense of family warmth and support, and gives the family itself a feeling of participation and usefulness. Once a nurse appreciates the complex feelings behind the relatives' behavior, she will have much more empathy, patience, and understanding.

ER: Are there any particular problems or areas of conflict concerning the nurse-patient-family relationship that occur more frequently than others?

FS: Yes. Some of the most difficult problems for the nurses revolve around the children of older patients. One often witnesses the culmination of long-term conflicts when a parent is seriously ill. A child who feels he has neglected his parents may try to compensate for this during the illness of one of them. He may externalize his guilty feelings by accusing the nursing staff of neglect. Obviously the nurses shouldn't take these accusations personally. They should understand that he is merely berating himself.

The family conflicts that surface in the hospital have usually been present for years, and a nurse would be naïve to think she could help solve them with a little attention and discussion. Child-parent conflicts can be deep and painful. Sometimes the parent perpetuates the suffering by refusing to accept his child's offer of help, saying "It's too late." The parent implies that he will carry his child's "crime" unexcused into the grave, and the child feels he can never atone for it. The nurse and the doctor must appreciate how powerful this experience can be and, when feasible, try to play the role of mediator. I have seen adult children engage in a fist fight in the hospital room when one accused another of not giving their parent the attention he needed.

ER: How else can a family create difficulties for the nursing staff?

FS: The family of terminally ill people can also be difficult if they have not accepted that their loved one is dying. This is hard on the patient, whose natural withdrawal into himself is contradicted by his relatives' refusal to let him die. This is more common when the patient is fairly young. The wife of a man in his forties, dying of advanced cancer, was so anxious about her husband that she woke him up every twenty minutes to find out his level of consciousness. She brought the children into the room and they prayed for an impossible recovery for hours each day. They prayed and cried for so long that when the end approached we had to bring in a special nurse to support them in case they became uncontrollable when he died. They did manage to cope with his death when it occurred, but their holding on made his dying more difficult for everyone, especially for him.

ER: Do you have any suggestions for achieving closer family cooperation with the hospital staff?

FS: A good way to sort out a lot of problems is for the doctor to call a family conference, and include the patient and the nursing staff. Then everyone is in the picture. Each knows what the other knows, and no one is being protected. It eliminates a lot of frustration. It eliminates pretense. A daughter needn't say, "Oh, mother, you're looking much better today," when both mother and daughter know she is actually looking a lot worse. Such a conference also provides the family with an opportunity to communicate directly with the doctor and the nursing staff. A nurse who is caring for a cancer patient becomes involved with the entire family, because the family and the patient go through the same agony.

ER: Mrs. Shepley, you've spoken of your involvement with your patients and of your own hurt when one of them suffers or dies. How does this affect your own family?

ES: My family is involved in my work. I talk about the problems of patients at home, because the patients are a part of my life. My family sympathizes with me when I need sympathy and supports me when I need support. When I go through a period of anxiety about a patient who has developed new metastases or a low blood count, my family suffers with me. I don't want to just be a clinical nurse while I'm in the hospital and then go home and forget about it. On the other hand, I don't let it dominate my life. I have plenty of activities and other involvements. I think that's very important.

ER: I wonder what all three of you feel about the limits of treatment. Should vigorous treatment ever be stopped, and when should it cease?

FS: I have strong feelings about that. The cessation of treatment is the doctor's decision, of course, but his decision affects the nursing staff. I have often seen a patient who is not responding to treatment. He may be breaking down with bedsores, mouth ulcers, and weight loss. Everything seems to be going against him, yet some doctors will still feel they must carry on treatment as vigorously as possible. Quite often I'll say, "For what? Why all this?" and the doctor may reply, "Well, there's always hope." I realize that no one wants to give up hope, but I feel that it would be better if doctors would get together with members of a family and say, "The time has come when we literally can do no more." However, some doctors seem to think the family's minds will be eased if the patient has a nasogastric tube and intravenous fluids. Also, I find that many doctors cannot accept death because they interpret it as a failure on their part. Many nurses also have difficulty in coping with a patient who is dying.

ES: A short time ago I helped care for a forty-five-year-old man who had recurrent colon cancer. He was on chemotherapy. We saw him once a week, and each time he was depressed, dependent, and totally dejected. Then one day his personality seemed to change. He sat up straight, seemed confident, and in a firm, clear voice announced that he didn't want any more chemotherapy, that it wasn't helping him, and that he was ready to die. He stated that he no longer liked his body and that he didn't like the kind of person he had become. He seemed relieved that he had reached this decision and had shared his feelings with me. His condition at that time was not really terminal, but to everyone's surprise, he was admitted to the hospital the following week with extreme weakness and died two days later.

I had asked him if he was frightened of a painful death because I wanted to reassure him that we could use medication to reduce his pain as much as possible. He said he was not afraid of pain, but that he didn't like the idea of IVs and other tubes. We also discussed his right to refuse treatment.

FS: I recently had a similar experience. I admitted a seventy-two-year-old patient with a leg ulcer. There was a form on the front of his chart which said that in the event of his having a heart attack, he did not want any heroics. He didn't want any cardiac resuscitation. He just wanted to be allowed to die in peace. That was the first form I've seen in this hospital, and I showed it to the staff. I said, "At last we're coming down to reality. Medical personnel are actually facing the fact that when the time comes, a patient should have the choice of how he is to die."

Peculiarly enough, the refusal of treatment is much more common in females than in males. They will say, "Oh, for goodness' sake, leave me alone. Let me die. Take that IV out." I'm sorry that in such a case my response must be, "You'll have to discuss this with your doctor." I have known two patients who said to their doctors point-blank, "I don't want any of this. Leave me alone."

ER: What did the doctors do in these cases?

FS: They had to accept their patients' wishes. A patient has the right to refuse treatment. Not long ago a patient with complete renal failure hadn't passed urine for a whole week. He had a cardiac problem as well as a malignancy. The doctor sat down to discuss the situation with me and said, "As far as I'm concerned there's nothing more we can do for this man." I said, "I wholeheartedly agree with you. We'll do what we can to make him comfortable." I came back the following day and the patient was again receiving intravenous fluids. When the doctor arrived, I asked him what had happened and he replied, "Believe it or not, his son said I had to continue the IVs." The patient lived four more days.

ML: People want to live, but everyone has his own set of conditions, and these conditions have to be respected. Some people would rather be dead than deformed or dependent. On the other hand, a lot of people sit around and say, "Boy, I wouldn't want anyone to have to do that for me." But if they become sick, they feel differently. Then they say, "I remember when I was well I thought I'd rather die than be in this condition. But now that I'm like this, I still want help. I still want to live." A patient has to be able to examine his own feelings, and we have to try to determine what he really wants.

ER: Patients often succeed in gaining extra time with a remission, but when this doesn't happen, I experience a sense of loss and defeat. How do you handle such feelings, Mrs. Shepley?

ES: I also feel helpless at times. However, everyone is going to die sometime or other, and there's not much I can do to alter that. If all I can do is help them through this difficult period, I feel I have accomplished something.

ER: Miss Lawton, do you think more people will become interested in going into oncology nursing, now that medical oncology has become a recognized subspecialty?

ML: Yes, especially if this leads to the creation of more cancer wards and cancer hospitals. Cancer used to be kept in the closet. The word was never used. I've seen old nursing textbooks full of tragic-sounding terminology that makes having cancer appear hopeless. We can throw those books away. There is hope.

16 · Social Service

Social workers who directly assist cancer patients are usually affiliated with hospitals, government agencies, or independent organizations such as the American Cancer Society. They evaluate, plan, coordinate resources, and support patients in a variety of ways, depending on the administrative structure and purposes of their organization. Their overall goals are the same—to help the cancer patient, emotionally, financially, and/or with material goods.

I interviewed two social workers in San Francisco. One is associated with the American Cancer Society; the other works with cancer patients at Mount Zion Hospital.*

THE AMERICAN CANCER SOCIETY

BARBARA KENT: As a social worker, my basic role is to assess clients' problems and work with them and their families. The difference for a social worker between working with cancer patients and with other clients lies in the knowledge she must have concerning certain problems that arise because of the nature of the disease. However, the basic approach is the same with all clients; you assess the family, the medical, financial, religious, and employment systems in which a person operates, and intervene appropriately with the individual, his family, or personnel in other agencies. You help people plan for their present and future, coordinate their resources, and deal with their feelings about their situation.

Cancer patients are referred to a social worker for many reasons: financial problems; care problems; problems they are having

* Barbara Kent, M.S.W., American Cancer Society, San Francisco; Assistant Service Director, Staff, Miller-Bunting Program for Cancer Patients; and Patricia Fobair, M.S.W., Claire Zellerbach Saroni Tumor Institute, Mount Zion Hospital and Medical Center.

with the institutions they are dealing with; problems they are having in understanding, or communicating with, their doctors; or emotional problems involving their personal lives.

Every referral comes to me at a point of crisis or stress. The first crisis may be the discovery of a symptom. Someone thinks, "I have a lump in my breast. Do I have cancer? Where can I get an exam? Now what can I do? What does this mean for my family?" If the disease progresses, there are other crises at various stages: recurrence, treatment, physical deterioration, dying, or death. Many of our referrals come from hospital social workers when the patient is about to return home after diagnostic work-up, surgery, radiation, chemotherapy treatment, or other acute problems.

Often a spouse who has been taking care of a wife or husband will phone for help when a problem arises that he or she cannot handle. The patient has become bedridden or incontinent, lost his job, has a recurrence of disease, or has in some way been forced to alter his role in the family. The focus of the crisis may be the family, the patient, or, more likely, a combination of the two. Part of my job is to try to decide where the problem lies and to assess the psychological state of the patient. His problem may not be caused by his present illness and crisis. However, most of the people we serve in our agency are psychologically "healthy people." But if my assessment is such that the patient or his family is not able to deal with the situation, I may say, "Let's get together on a regular basis," or I may say nothing and simply contact them regularly. There are some kinds of crises, the ones I just mentioned, that are predictable. This means that if I hear about changes that may increase stress, I can intervene at the right time. If my assessment reveals that the person has not functioned well in the past and may not function well in his new situation, I may provide brief psychotherapy myself, or, more usually, I refer him to an appropriate community agency.

The psychotherapeutic counseling that I give or arrange is usually aimed at a reduction of anxiety or depression, the restoration of hope, and the desensitization of trauma. For example, if a patient goes into the hospital, I may phone the hospital social worker and ask her to stop by to see how he is doing, check his clinical status, and let me know when he is going home. When a patient goes into the hospital and I have been working with him very closely, I stop by frequently to say hello. I may see a patient at home once a month, or every two weeks, or just talk to him on the phone. Flexibility is an important part of my job.

As assistant service director in the American Cancer Society, I am also partly responsible for several ongoing programs: an informational-referral-assistive program; a transportation program;

and the rehabilitation programs—Reach to Recovery, the Lost Chord Club, and the Ostomy Association.*

The American Cancer Society provides an information referral service to patients. Our unit gets about two thousand calls a year, asking such questions as, "Will you please send me some literature? Where can I get a breast exam? Where can I get a pap test?" Sometimes more than a simple answer is required. If you ask why the person wants to know, you discover that the caller has a lump and is worried about it, or that there is some other troubling symptom. Such a call may turn into a brief counseling session, or the person who answers the telephone may tell the caller, "You seem upset; would you like to talk to the social worker?" and transfer the call to me.

Another service we provide is sickroom and patient-care equipment, which we call assistive devices. We lend common things such as wheelchairs, walkers, commodes, bedpans, and canes. In addition, we may provide prosthetic devices such as breast prostheses for women with mastectomies, electrolarynxes for laryngectomy patients, wigs for people who lose their hair, colostomy equipment, ileostomy equipment, or little things like surgical tape. We really try to provide whatever the patient needs.

ER: Many patients may not be able to afford these devices after they've paid their other medical bills.

BK: That's right. Fortunately there are a variety of sources of help. We investigate these possible sources of assistance, and if we find none of them is available for a particular patient, then we supply him with whatever he needs.

ER: Does the ACS help cancer patients defray the cost of transportation to and from treatment?

BK: Yes. In San Francisco the ACS sponsors a transportation program that primarily uses taxis. The first priority is given to patients who have daily radiation treatment. The second priority is for people who have weekly chemotherapy, or some other kind of regular treatment. People who go to the doctor for periodic follow-ups or checkups are referred to other resources for help with transportation.

ER: Isn't transporting patients to and from treatment something volunteers could do?

BK: We do have some volunteers, but not nearly enough. We

* Reach to Recovery is discussed later in this book. Those who want more information about the other programs, or about the chapter nearest them, should write to the United Ostomy Associaion, 1111 Wilshire Boulevard, Los Angeles, California 90017, or the International Association of Laryngectomies, 219 East Forty-second Street, New York, N. Y., 10017.

have not been successful in developing a volunteer driver program in San Francisco.

ER: There is also a unique program available to cancer patients in San Francisco. Could you describe it?

BK: The San Francisco unit of the American Cancer Society is unique in having the Miller-Bunting Program for Cancer Patients. This program has been invaluable to cancer patients. We receive a grant of $100,000 a year from the San Francisco Foundation. The total amount is used for patient reimbursement of expenses. A community advisory committee sets policy and evaluates the program. The Cancer Society provides the administrative and personnel costs of the program. The grant specifies that social work assistance in planning and counseling must be provided for recipients of funds.

Right now we use about one-third of the money for maintenance. This provides monies for room and board for people out of the area who need treatment in San Francisco. These patients are always referred to us by hospital social workers, who provide us with the appropriate medical and casework histories, and with ongoing casework for the patients receiving funds. In these cases we serve as consultant and fiscal agent.

The other two uses of the grant money are attendant care and chemotherapy needs. Attendant care is loosely defined; it can mean anything from heavy housework to personal care twenty-four hours a day. The purpose is to help keep a patient at home as long as he wishes. We reimburse him for these costs. The attendants are people who will come regularly, without fail, and who have experience with cancer patients. Nothing fazes them; they come in and take over. They provide food, and give personal care. The family immediately relaxes, yet all I have done is provide that needed help.

The Miller-Bunting Program also helps people who have had a mastectomy or a hysterectomy, and who may only need a week or two of help to get back on their feet when they go home after surgery.

ER: Are the attendants employed by the Cancer Society?

BK: No. They are independent contractors. We maintain a list of people who like to work with cancer patients and who have been found to be good with them. We also refer patients who need attendants to home care agencies; at other times they may find their own attendants. Most attendant referrals come from hospitals, but many also come from the patients themselves, their families, friends, and physicians. All referrals are assessed by the social work staff during a home visit, and plans are made in consultation with the doctor, and/or a registered nurse.

Chemotherapy referrals come primarily from physicians who are familiar with the fact that we can pay for some drugs and laboratory work.

ER: Many patients referred to me have incurred extensive medical expenses from either surgery or radiotherapy, sometimes from both. They may not be qualified for the Medicare or the MediCal program, but at the same time they need financial aid. Some of the highest costs in treating cancer are the drugs, laboratory tests, and X rays. The Miller-Bunting Program for Cancer Patients has been of great value and support to all the patients I've referred to you.

BK: I think the chemotherapists have found that this is a useful program for their patients. Of course, every time we accept a chemotherapy patient we hope the drugs are going to be effective and keep him alive a long, long time; maintenance may therefore continue for years. Every time we add a case we are making a potential long-term commitment.

ER: Are you sometimes forced to turn down the requests of older people or people who do not have families to support because you have limited funds?

BK: We haven't yet had to face that problem. We evaluate a patient's total family situation and consider a number of factors, such as resources versus expenditures, family composition, debts, the stage of diagnosis, and the possibility of going back to work. We have been able to use flexible guidelines. Generally, the program helps those who "fall between the cracks," that is, those who are not eligible for a welfare program but who also are not wealthy. We also evaluate many people who need never receive financial aid from us because we find they are eligible for other programs in the community. We help them get assistance from these resources.

A lot of patients won't say to their doctor, "I am having trouble paying for this." They're afraid the doctor will stop treating them. Some doctors feel that it's not appropriate for them to discuss finances with their patients. Thus they never ask them whether they are having difficulty paying for their treatment.

ER: In other words, a limited number of physicians are referring patients to the program for assistance.

BK: That's right, and I would therefore like to encourage doctors to use the social worker as part of the team. Some doctors don't seem to have the inclination or the time to look beyond the disease and treatment to the total problems of the patient. Others say, "It's not my province." The social worker, on the other hand, does have a certain area of expertise, which I define as the process of looking at the *whole* situation and trying to identify the problem.

I have a patient of yours who needs reassurance about her medical condition. She defines what I do for her as "translating what the doctor tells me." I am cautious about that because I may not know the medical situation; so whenever she asks specific medical questions, I encourage her to go back to you for clarification.

ER: This lady, a refugee who was in a concentration camp, is approximately fifty years old, and has developed breast cancer. She feels that taking chemotherapy is almost worse than being in a concentration camp. She has suppressed this past experience. Her current fear is of death, and this fear has made her afraid of therapy. She is a nonbeliever who wants to believe and needs reassurance. How have you handled her?

BK: I have seen her several times and have observed a change in her emotional status. She had never really worked through her feelings about the mastectomy she had three years ago. She just hoped she would never have to deal with cancer again. It is something inside of her that she can't see and can't feel. She doesn't know whether the cancer is growing, or whether the treatment is working, or is going to work. She has always coped with her problems in an intellectual way. By the time of my second visit she had read a lot about cancer and was trying to understand all the information she had acquired. Initially she was concerned because she had been referred to a new doctor whom she didn't know. She was unable to trust him as she had trusted her former doctor. I encouraged her to accept the new doctor on the strength of the recommendation of her trusted physician. We quickly established a rapport because she felt I could understand her. I think she is a religious woman who derives strength from that. I'm not sure how much emotional support she gets from her family, although she can turn to them for concrete needs. She is basically a strong woman who has survived a great deal. I've supported her by saying, "Look, you've done this before." Also, like many other people, she feels that cancer has never happened to anyone else. When I say to her, "I know other people who have gotten this treatment," it helps instill the feeling that she's not alone. Many patients derive a similar feeling of shared experience when they participate in one of the discussion groups that are organized especially for cancer patients.

ER: Have you worked with any patients who have not been told they have cancer?

BK: We do work with some patients who do not know they have cancer. In these cases I am introduced as a social worker, referred by whoever seems appropriate. I have also participated in family discussions in which a patient is finally told he has cancer.

I also work with many terminally ill patients. We talk about their feelings about dying and the emotional consequences their death will have on their families; and we deal with practical matters, such as arranging for the custody of children or planning funerals.

ER: Are you in touch with other social workers who deal with cancer patients?

BK: Yes. We now have an oncology social workers' group that meets once a month. We have been sharing our mutual concerns and attempting to assist other social workers who deal with cancer patients. The group meets under the auspices of the National Association of Social Workers. The Cancer Society also sponsors workshops for social workers, in which I participate.

ER: How would you summarize your role?

BK: The primary function of every social worker is to assess the total needs of a patient and to suggest ways in which to meet those needs. Within the medical system we may work with the doctors, support the patient during medical treatment, or assist the patient in his negotiations with medical personnel. Within the family system we may help the family cope with the emotional aspects of their cancer problems as well as the concrete problems created by the disease process. Sometimes we become involved in the patient's dealings with the welfare and/or school system or assist in re-employment.

There are two things that I say to all patients and their families: "I will be here as long as you need me," which includes the time following the death of the patient, if the family needs me; and I also tell them, "I can't cure your cancer and I can't keep you alive. Now what is it we can do?" We recognize the realities of living with cancer and then try to work on those areas over which we have control. Sometimes I provide very concrete items that make patients more comfortable. Fortunately, I have these at my disposal.

Also, the fact that I am identified as a representative of the American Cancer Society makes talking to me about cancer immediately acceptable. A patient and/or his family and I can then deal with the fears and fantasies of cancer and death.

ER: You have the patient's cooperation because you have something to give. It's tangible; it's not just lip service.

STAFF-PATIENT DISCUSSION GROUP, CLAIRE ZELLERBACH SARONI
TUMOR INSTITUTE, MOUNT ZION HOSPITAL AND MEDICAL CENTER

PATRICIA FOBAIR: The first meeting of the staff-patient discussion group at the Claire Zellerbach Saroni Institute took place in February 1972. The idea for forming the group came to me when I noticed that a number of patients were lingering around the Institute after completing their course of radiation therapy. Though their disease was in remission, they seemed lost; they didn't know what to do with themselves. I thought they might need to talk about what that meant in terms of present strain and worry.

At an Institute staff meeting I introduced the idea of bringing these patients together with staff members for informal discussions. A resident and two staff members were willing to participate on a trial basis, so the first meeting consisted of these three people, six or seven patients, and myself.

ER: How did that first group of patients respond to the experience?

PF: They came to the meeting because they liked the idea, but they were also apprehensive. They didn't know exactly what was going to happen, and they weren't certain that they wanted therapy sessions. However, they soon relaxed and began to talk.

They first discussed their angry feelings toward their physicians. They vented a lot of anger about what had happened to them during their diagnostic and treatment periods. Later they discussed problems in their personal lives. These were usually related to employment, family relationships, and the broader issue of their own mental health.

ER: What did you feel were the sources of their anger, especially toward their physicians?

PF: There were several factors. Some patients were angry at themselves for having acquired the disease. They felt their bodies had let them down. They couldn't understand this or answer the question, "Why me?" Others were angry because there had been a delay in obtaining a diagnosis. Whether this was their own fault or that of a doctor, the resulting frustration had to be integrated with their other feelings.

Several of the patients had problems that originated in the doctor-patient relationship. A doctor is in a position of great importance, a God-like figure. Few patients feel themselves to be his peers. Instead, they have toward doctors some of the parent-child feelings that accompany reverence for authority. The patients in the group needed a chance to reassert themselves and equalize the score. Being a patient meant submitting to medical care and going along with someone else's program, and they were reluctant to do that without offering some resistance. Their entire medical experience was a regressive one that they were partly able to overcome by releasing emotional tension in the group discussions.

ER: The group was successful, then, in helping them to think through their problems. How did they actually accomplish this? What steps were involved?

PF: They went through a number of stages. They began, as I said, by telling their medical stories and talking about their unhappy feelings. After a few weeks they were less depressed. Then they began to talk about their personal problems. They got a lot of support from the other members of the group and they soon began to take more responsibility for directing their lives in areas over which they had some control. For example, a widowed lady with ovarian cancer used the group for one year. She had had a distressing surgical experience at another hospital and was able to reveal her feelings about that, the hospital staff, and her disease. Eventually she began to talk about her relationships with her son and daughter, and the difficulties the three of them had shared after the death of her husband. She also discussed her relationship with her sister, whom she had always envied. After sharing her feelings about these experiences for several weeks, she suddenly began to talk about her hobbies and interests and about new activities in which she might participate. Within a year of joining the group, she had planned and successfully taken a trip to Europe, changed her place of living, and started a new life.

ER: Did some patients fail to benefit from the group, and, if so, to what do you attribute their failure to use the group to their advantage?

PF: Over a period of months and years there have been patients who entered the group in the hope of finding something for themselves but who discovered they could not work out their problems or get support from the other patients. To try to find out why this occurred, I developed a questionnaire that I circulated to all the patient participants. I've observed that if a patient comes into the group when he is very sick or in a deeply depressed state of mind and does not find someone else in the group with whom to identify, he finds it difficult to make a connection with the group as a whole. A group tends to operate on the basis of identification among its members and the projection of one's own problems onto others. Also, some people choose to withdraw at critical moments in their lives rather than to talk about their problems. But I've discovered that people who are willing to talk, and who use talking as a way of relating to others and solving problems, get the most out of this kind of therapy.

The willingness to speak about having cancer is also important, but not all patients feel it is helpful to communicate openly about their disease process. They feel that it will seem worse if they talk too much about it, and they prefer to try to put it out of their minds between treatments.

Some patients have such strong emotional support within their families and such good prognoses that they have no need for the group.

ER: Do you think that some patients who don't feel they benefit from the group are people who are failing medically and who expected the group to solve some of their medical problems?

PF: Yes. It's common for a patient to have a fantasy that the group can solve his medical problems. He will say, "I wish the doctor . . ." or "I wish the group could solve my cancer problems."

Our group is composed of 50 percent patients with cures or good remissions and 50 percent patients with progressive disease. The latter patients joined the group when they knew they were not doing well medically but when they were still active physically and eager to participate in group discussions. Later, when they became weaker, and showed physical deterioration, they were able to use the group for support. Quite a few of them died while still members of the group.

ER: How do the other members of the group feel and how do they behave when such a person is failing?

PF: They feel very sad. It's important, in a group process, for members to share with the failing member their own feelings about his impending death and to ask him how he wants them to act.

This is happening in the group right now. A patient with rectal carcinoma that has metastasized has used the group as a source of energy and a means of maintaining his activity level. He's a person who believes in communicating. Now that he's going downhill, he is asked by the others at the beginning of many of our sessions how he wants us to respond to him. Does he want us to ignore the fact that he's failing or does he want us to talk about it and give him feedback? He says he wants us to be honest and direct with him, and he also is able to let us express our feelings for him. However, when I told him I was sad about the way he looked, he said, "I'll forgive you this time, but I really don't want you to feel sad for me." He still wants people to feel as though he is going to make it and to help bolster him. I suspect that should this particular patient die, a number of us will go to his funeral because of the intensity of our feelings for him. We've also been involved with his family because his wife and children have used the group.

ER: Do the families of patients participate in the group?

PF: Yes, quite a few spouses come. It's up to a patient to invite his or her spouse and the spouse is free to accept or decline the invitation. The group is very open-ended that way.

ER: What is the average number of participants in the group?

PF: We average eight to fourteen patients, plus two or three staff members, per session. We've had as many as seventeen to twenty patients at one time, but that has proved unwieldy. We meet once a week for two hours.

ER: How many relatives usually come?

PF: It fluctuates. The maximum number of relatives who have attended a particular session has been three. Right now there are only one or two.

ER: Have you heard of groups similar to yours in any other part of the United States?

PF: The first group I heard about before ours was at the University of California Medical School in the maxillo-facial unit, where Doris Ordway had a group for cancer patients who had undergone head or neck surgery. Since then I've been told about groups at Memorial Hospital in New York that consist of postoperative mastectomy patients and their relatives. Stanford University Hospital has a group especially for new cancer patients and a group for patients with advanced breast cancer. Other groups are being formed in San Francisco. Kaiser Hospital has started a group that is attended by a social worker, an oncology nurse, and a psychologist.

I think our group is unique because it includes patients with different diagnoses, ages, stages of disease, and family situations. Also, we focus on rehabilitation. A patient in our group is encouraged to do all he can to adjust to his disease and not let it ruin his life.

ER: In other words, you are helping patients to develop a way of life rather than an approach to death.

PF: Yes, but we do discuss death, of course. Nevertheless, the group is most valuable in helping people to live with their disease. The patients have defined this as their focus and I certainly concur. Their attitude is, "First you mourn and grieve your condition and then you figure out what you can do to improve your life."

The group is a place for patients to talk over the problems of cancer that affect daily living. We encourage them to be frank with their doctors and not to let the hospital, as an institution, get the best of them. They are encouraged to defend themselves, to fight if an employer lays them off their job; and, if they do not succeed in such a situation, to find new employment.

ER: How would you summarize the value of the group to the patients who participate, and what are your plans for the future?

PF: I learned from the questionnaire that patients slept better, were less depressed, and were able to talk about their illness with greater comfort as a result of being in the group for several months. The group is therefore one of several possible means by which patients can become more comfortable with what is essentially a stress situation. Because of our success, we hope to establish more groups in the future, including one for younger patients, and perhaps one for spouses.

ER: Are you doing anything to assist the family after the death of one of your patients?

PF: So far that is an unmet need.

ER: I am organizing a group called the Helping Hand to help support people who are grieving. The purpose of the Helping Hand will be to have someone who has been through the grieving and recovery period help a person who is in the process of grieving.

17 · Volunteers

Volunteers, like social workers, nurses, and clergymen, must be sensitive to the needs of the people they serve. Their goal is to complement the skills of these professionals and to offer patients one more means of emotional or tangible support. Their efforts can often fill a need for nonmedical support to aid in a patient's recovery. Volunteers who work with cancer patients may have a specific, clearly defined goal, as the women who work for the American Cancer Society's Reach to Recovery Program do, or they may function within flexible guidelines, like those who have joined the Patient Service program at Mount Zion Hospital. This chapter contains excerpts from interviews with a former volunteer executive of the Reach to Recovery Program and with volunteers in the Patient Service program.*

THE REACH TO RECOVERY PROGRAM OF THE AMERICAN CANCER SOCIETY†

ER: In 1969 the Reach to Recovery Program became affiliated nationally with the American Cancer Society. You helped organize that program in California and served as Volunteer Coordinator for the state from 1969 to 1974. How did you become interested in Reach to Recovery?

RHODA GOLDMAN: Nineteen years ago I had a mastectomy. While

---

* Rhoda Goldman, Volunteer Coordinator, Reach to Recovery Program, American Cancer Society; San Francisco Unit: 1968–present; California Division: 1969–74; and Shirley Selby, chairman, and Laura Williams, volunteer since 1971, in the Patient Service Department, Department of Volunteers, Mount Zion Hospital and Medical Center.

† The American Cancer Society also sponsors a rehabilitation visiting program for ostomy patients and cooperates with similar programs of the United Ostomy Association and the Lost Chord Club of the International Association of Laryngectomies. For addresses, see the footnote on page 160.

I was in the hospital I received visits from two friends who had had the same operation. I could see that they had resumed normal lives, and that gave me courage. I am now convinced that the only people who can offer that kind of encouragement and inspire that kind of confidence are women who have had similar experiences.

Sometime after my surgery I became aware of the Reach to Recovery Program through a friend of one of the founders,* and events moved from there.

ER: What is the primary message carried by volunteers of Reach to Recovery to women who have just undergone mastectomies?

RG: Our message is that there is no reason you cannot continue your former life-style exactly as it was before surgery. You should not think of yourself as different or as a person apart from the community.

ER: Can anyone who has had a mastectomy become a volunteer?

RG: No. We screen our volunteers very carefully and train them under professional supervision. I think this is one of the strongest points of the program. This means that a woman who visits a new mastectomy patient doesn't just go into her room and say, "I've had a mastectomy and look at how well I'm doing. Everything is going to be fine with you." On the contrary, in the training sessions volunteers are taught what they should and should not say. For instance, they never discuss medical matters. They urge a patient to save those questions for her physician. However, they can relieve a lot of anxiety by answering the many small questions that have begun to loom very large. They are taught to think in terms of an individual's needs and to offer advice that is appropriate and supportive for a particular person. We try to match them in terms of personal experience, particularly with regard to age and marital status.

ER: How many times does a volunteer visit a patient?

RG: A volunteer makes one visit, which she follows up with a telephone call. This is usually sufficient for most patients. We are wary of creating a dependent relationship on the part of a patient toward a volunteer, or vice versa. Occasionally a further visit or telephone call can be made where advisable, upon request.

ER: Does that mean that most doctors support your program?

RG: Most, but not all. Some physicians have resisted using our services, even though the California Medical Association has approved the Reach to Recovery Program. These physicians who resist may do it out of ignorance of our goals or through fear that

* Reach to Recovery was originated by Terese Lasser in 1952.

a visit by a nonprofessional will cause emotional disturbance to their patient. They may also just be concerned about interference in the doctor-patient relationship.

One thing we are trying to do that may help win physician support is to arrange that Reach to Recovery have a base in each hospital. A liaison person in the hospital would contact a Reach to Recovery volunteer whenever a mastectomy is performed. This would not only insure that each mastectomy patient would have the benefit of a visit from a volunteer but that the visit would be made at the ideal time, which we have found to be between the third and sixth postoperative days. A visit during that period seems to offer the most encouragement and to stimulate the strongest desire for a good future adjustment.

ER: How well do you think most women adjust to a mastectomy?

RG: I'd say that over 90 percent make a very good adjustment. We encourage a woman to face it, cope with it, and do whatever she can to help herself to recover. We tell her that her family and friends will take their cue from the way she reacts. She is encouraged to discuss her thoughts and emotions with those close to her.

Sometimes there is a need for further counseling, however, either for the woman herself or for a member of her family. For instance, a husband can often benefit from talking to someone about his own and his wife's feelings toward the mastectomy. The adjustment of the husband or children, other family members or friends is very important to a woman's recovery. Therefore, the availability of counseling for all these people is an essential of good care. For this reason, a volunteer will often ask a woman, "Would you like us to talk to your husband too?" or "How is your husband taking it?"

ER: What is the most prevalent fear among women faced with the possibility of a mastectomy?

RG: A lot of people are afraid they will be mutilated. The fear of mutilation is strong because our society is so breast-conscious. Women worry about their future sex lives. We have created an image of the physically perfect woman, and a woman facing a mastectomy thinks, "I won't match up any more." That is why we emphasize in our Reach to Recovery literature that femininity and womanliness aren't dependent on a few ounces of flesh.

Considering the trauma that most women undergo in having a mastectomy, I think that some kind of preoperative consultation should take place with the doctor. For that matter, there should be a dialogue between a doctor and his patient before any kind of surgery, even before a biopsy, so that people can be helped to face reality.

ER: I agree. Such discussions would remove some of the fear of the unknown. We also need to attack the fear that women have of self-examination and the possibility of discovering a lump. Does the Reach to Recovery Program do anything to encourage self-examination of the breasts?

RG: Those of us within the program have been advocating the adoption of such a policy for years. I feel it would give the program an added dimension if Reach to Recovery volunteer visitors were among those who participate in teaching breast self-examination. The willingness of Mrs. Ford and Mrs. Rockefeller to share their experiences with American women not only saved many lives by encouraging women to examine themselves and consult their physicians, but they helped bring the whole subject out into the open. Too many women in the past have felt ashamed and wanted to conceal the fact that they had had mastectomies. In my own case it was basically a matter of life or death. There was never any question about the operation. I received the very best treatment and was given a lot of emotional support by my doctor, family, and friends. I never felt ashamed, and I never felt it was a deterrent. On the contrary, I think I'm basically a better person for it. This is the way I am, and the important fact is that I'm living today and leading an active, involved, and satisfying life.

ER: What is your hope for mastectomy patients in the future?

RG: I hope that in the future everyone who has a mastectomy will receive a visit from a Reach to Recovery volunteer, since our primary concern is for the quality of life after surgery.

THE PATIENT SERVICE DEPARTMENT, MOUNT ZION HOSPITAL AND MEDICAL CENTER

Most hospitals have an active volunteer corps of men and women. The Department of Volunteers at Mount Zion Hospital has developed a unique program called Patient Service. It offers volunteers a way of serving patients that requires an unusual degree of tact, sensitivity, and emotional fortitude.

One of the originators of the program as it exists today was a former patient, Shirley Selby, who wanted to share with other patients the good will and kindness she felt she received during her hospitalization. The original concept behind Patient Service was to provide a number of small services and extra comforts for patients. This would also benefit nurses and other medical personnel by freeing them for work that required their special training.

Since 1969 the program has been expanded in personnel and scope.

In 1970 the director of volunteers* organized a series of seminars at which the needs of cancer patients were discussed by the appropriate professionals and the volunteers.

More recently, in the fall of 1974, I added to the Patient Service program by initiating a series of monthly noontime meetings that are attended not only by volunteers but by any other interested hospital staff—nurses, social workers, and interns. The meetings are informal. Speakers range from the patients themselves to experienced professionals. These people share their experiences and talk about particular problems of cancer patients.

ER: Mrs. Selby, how does a person become a member of Patient Service?

SHIRLEY SELBY: Prospective volunteers are first screened by the director or the assistant director of volunteers. If they appear qualified for, and interested in, the Patient Service Department, they are referred to me for a further interview. The particular qualities we seek in new volunteers are awareness and sensitivity to others, the ability to listen, flexibility, and a willingness to be objective and nonjudgmental. New Patient Service volunteers receive extensive training from those who are already in the program, the length of training varying according to the experience of the individual. They are advised how to ask and reply to the questions of seriously ill people and cautioned against making any attempt to discuss present or future prognoses.

ER: What do Patient Service volunteers actually do, Mrs. Williams?

LAURA WILLIAMS: Most volunteers spend only one or two days a week at the hospital. On arrival we go to the nurse on the floor to which we've been assigned and ask the nurse what special tasks need to be done that day. During the time we spend at the hospital we may accompany patients to X ray, relay messages from patients to nurses, feed patients (only at the request of the nurse), run errands for the patients or the nurses, take care of patients' flowers, or change their drinking water. We also just visit with patients. Volunteers play card games, do crossword puzzles, read out loud, discuss anything from the patient's feelings about his disease and his treatment to politics and baseball. Or we may silently hold a hand, or sit quietly and listen.

Listening to a patient is the most important thing we do. It helps us more than anything else to gain understanding. We learn to interpret subtle changes in mood or train of thought. Often, by the time a volunteer has performed some simple task she will be

* Mrs. Frank Culp, former director of volunteers, Mount Zion Hospital and Medical Center.

able to determine whether a patient wants to talk or has an unspoken need. An anxious look may reveal whether the patient is saying, "I don't feel like a visit today," or "I want to tell you something." Sometimes it is simply the wrong moment to approach a patient. Sometimes the volunteer is the wrong person to make such an approach. The members of Patient Service recognize that, because of personality differences, they will not be acceptable to every patient, and they are aware that another volunteer may succeed in comforting a patient where they have failed.

ER: Mrs. Selby, do you discuss medical information with a patient?

SS: Patient Service volunteers feel it is neither necessary nor appropriate for them to have medical information concerning the patients they serve. They never ask for, and they are rarely given, any details of a patient's condition or medical treatment. This policy is in accord with our desire to offer help to all patients, not just those with cancer. Whoever the patient, whatever he tells us, our only concern is to listen compassionately and nonjudgmentally.

Patient confidences are respected at all times. Volunteers are told many things of a personal nature that could later be an embarrassment to a patient. The only possible occasion when a volunteer might repeat something told him by a patient is when the information is pertinent to that patient's care and recovery. The information is then relayed to the proper source—the nurse. For example, a patient may have a minor physical complaint, such as indigestion, that he did not consider worth mentioning to the nurse, but which he may have mentioned to us. We are therefore in a position to help the patient by telling the nurse, who can quickly provide relief.

ER: What do you consider the most important factor in achieving success with a program like Patient Service, Mrs. Williams?

LW: We recognize that the success of our program has depended on one thing: winning the confidence and respect of the nursing staff.

ER: You have been invaluable to both the nurses and the patients. From my own experience I know that the most important need of a patient, after medical care, is the availability of a sympathetic listener.

18 · The Clergy

Men and women of the clergy occupy a unique position. Whether Protestant ministers, Catholic priests, or Jewish rabbis, they have authority and respect in the community. One of their many functions is to comfort the sick, at home or in the hospital. The patients they visit in a hospital are not necessarily limited to members of one congregation, or even one religion. Some patients may no longer have any religious affiliation. Yet the clergy can still be welcome figures, sympathetic listeners, sources of emotional and spiritual sustenance.

Many people under the stress of illness or dying call upon God to help them. Severe stress and fear may also cause them to revert to previously held religious views. For these people, as well as for regular members of church, temple, or synagogue, the clergyman represents faith, salvation, and the authority of God. He is expected to have special insight into the mysteries of life and death.

I interviewed representatives of three faiths—Chaplain Laursen, Father Shanahan, and Rabbi Asher*—to ask them how they approached individual patients and how those patients reacted to them. What follows is not a comprehensive discussion of religion; it is an attempt to understand the role of the clergy with regard to the patient who has cancer. In spite of the many differences among the three faiths, in both concept and practice, I found that in dealing with the cancer patient the three clergymen differed only in style. Their objectives were similar—to help people to live, and also to die. In this respect their roles do not differ from those of doctors, nurses, social workers, and volunteers.

* The Reverend Elmer Laursen, D.Min., Chaplain and Supervisor, Clinical Pastoral Education, University of California, San Francisco; the Reverend John D. Shanahan, formerly Roman Catholic Chaplain, UCSF, presently Pastor, Star of the Sea Church, Sausalito; and Rabbi Joseph Asher, Temple Emanuel, San Francisco.

JOHN SHANAHAN: There are, of course, certain expectations, somewhat vaguely conceived, of what a clergyman should do. He is expected to minister to the patient, to provide the opportunity for sacraments and prayer, to bring comfort and solace in some way, to deal with spiritual problems, to lift the patient's morale, and to spread comfort and cheer. In the popular dichotomy, the doctor cares for the body, the chaplain cares for the soul. The clergyman has the opportunity to make a unique and valuable contribution to the spiritual, mental, and emotional well-being of the sick, the seriously ill, and the dying.

As a priest in a hospital setting, I am, among other things, acting as a representative of our religious community. The patients don't know me personally. They come from various parts of the Bay Area. They are separated from their families. My being there says, "We care about you. We want you to get well. How can we help?" Maybe these people haven't seen a priest in a long time. But my presence might remind them of a time when they attended church and thereby give them strength for the present. On the other hand, some people with tenuous ties to our religious community don't care about seeing a priest, so my visit to them will not be supportive. Each patient reacts differently. Therefore I don't have a planned approach.

Slowly and painfully I have learned one general approach. I think this approach helps me, as a priest caring for the seriously ill, to listen, and I hope it has helped the patients I visit. Unaware of the dynamics behind the emotional stresses or moral disorders in a man about to die, with not the faintest idea of what to say, I listen. I have learned to hold my tongue, learned what not to say. I try to show sincere interest, to reflect understanding of the person's feelings. I try to accept the man as a fellow human being. As a listener, I have learned that I can create an atmosphere of solicitous permissiveness in which the troubled patient feels free to share the burden he is unable to carry alone. I try to be compassionate, to touch the emotional pulse of the patient by identifying in some personal way with his anguish, his bewilderment, his interior conflict. I try to understand. I need hardly say a word. Someone is interested; someone understands; someone is in no hurry to run, to belittle, to disparage or explain away the worry or trot out pious cliches. I am, primarily, a listener whose contribution is a wholehearted acceptance of the patient. I try to create a climate in which the sick man feels he may speak without fear.

JOSEPH ASHER: I feel that my function is to try to be an empathic person who relates to people not as a rabbi but as a friend. The only rabbinic component of this kind of relationship is that perhaps the person has more respect and regard for me because he recognizes that I have seen other people in his same situation and

may even have some direct communication with the divine. But I
don't have that. I really don't think I have ever contributed to a
person to the extent that I have evoked resources of strength he
did not have before I came. The best I have been able to do is
maybe to awaken resources which this person was planning to set
aside or was unaware he possessed.

I may say to a patient, "Now look, every day that you live is
one more opportunity for an improvement in your condition, because with medical science the way it is today, what is impossible
today may be possible tomorrow." I also explain to him that much
of survival, and this may be impression rather than fact, depends
on a person's will and a person's desire to survive.

Recently a member of my congregation had a stroke and simply
did not want to live. He would not participate in such therapy as
was available to him and after a period of months he just died.
The physician who took care of him told me that this man could
have lived longer and could have lived an active life. This man simply did not want to live. So what I can do, as a rabbi, is constantly
reassure a patient that a great deal of his recovery depends on his
will to live. If I can help strengthen that will to live, I have made a
contribution.

Nevertheless, I'm terribly aware of my impotence in these things.
It's very difficult for an outside force to have any effect in a situation like this. People's lives cannot be influenced to such an extent
that a person can say, "The rabbi was here and he told me I'm
going to live. Therefore I'm going to live. I'm going to try harder
than I did before he came in." The person may do this for five
minutes, in my presence, but if his nature is inclined toward giving
up, that's what he's going to do.

However, I think we often underestimate both patients' ability
to cope and their need for comfort arising from an apprehension
of the truth. We always think they need to be babied when they
are in such situations. It is really more the function of the rabbi to
relate to the family, to help them accept the inevitable with grace
and with a certain amount of consolation. They in turn convey this
composure to the sick person. The entire Jewish tradition teaches
us to confront reality. If a person is about to die, then we have to
recognize the fact that this is about to happen. We do not, under
any circumstances, encourage a kind of covering up of what is
about to occur, nor do we hold out a description of a life beyond.
That is why it's sometimes much more difficult for a rabbi to comfort a family, particularly when a death occurs that is out of the
ordinary. In such instances the family's first response is often,
"How could God let this happen to us? What justice is there from
such a God?" I tell them that God is not doing something to hurt
them. The untimely death of the person they love is simply one of
the malfunctions of nature to which we are exposed from time to

time. Death before one's time is a malfunction of nature just as much as an earthquake or a hurricane.

ELMER LAURSEN: Patients have fear of cancer as a disease, and they need to share their fear and anxiety with someone who will listen. Many physicians and nurses listen to patients, but a clergyman may do it in a different way. He comes to listen to their questions, which often include "Why did this happen? What did I do?"

Our objective is to support patients in the most appropriate way. We try to keep hope alive, but not to foster false hope. We share the bad times that depress patients. We try to help them accept illness as a part of their life instead of just to fight it. We try to emphasize the positives in their lives, but when there are few or none of these it is harder to help them.

I attempt to console and share and be alongside of people during their suffering. I listen to their questions in a supportive way, helping them tap and enlarge upon their religious resources. I listen, and sometimes in silence I give aid and comfort. Frequently my main function is just to be there. I try to hear patients' verbal and nonverbal cries and concerns and, if possible, to help them achieve a new perspective. It seems to me that by sharing I contribute the important element, which is to help them feel less alone and less deserted.

When there are family members, relatives, and friends who are a part of the supportive system for a patient, I can at times also help them with their feelings and enable them to be supportive rather than hindering to the patient.

I have become increasingly aware that in our work with people and their problems, we need not pretend to have any great answers for them. They sometimes find answers for themselves, or at the least they find someone with whom they can share their questions.

While as a chaplain my desire is to work closely with the physician, he is not always ready to involve me in patient care. Often I am able to minister effectively in spite of his reluctance to include me. However, we both do a better job when we can work together.

The acceptance of the problem of illness and the incorporation of that acceptance into one's life and trying to deal with it is a process, an upward process. People who learn to accept and reconcile themselves to dying often seem to live more effectively. Given the opportunity to vent their anger at God in the presence of an understanding clergyman, they may be relieved of their guilt feelings. It is normal to be angry, curse, or swear at God and ask, "Why?" Eventually they learn that they can be as angry as they wish at God because He is big enough to handle it. Then they can begin a more dynamic process of living for their remaining time.

Somehow, it is helpful to most of us to be able to accept that death is a part of life.

The process of learning how best to support a patient is long and arduous. It involves going into a patient's room, letting him say whatever he wishes, and then helping him to look at what is going on, to reflect on it. I feel it is unnecessary to confront a person too heavily or bluntly. I have better ways of being with a patient than saying, "You know, you have to take a look at this for your wife and family. You can't just give up." Rather, I try to help him take hold of the problem and deal openly with it.

Finally, the time arrives when all I can do is to help a patient to die graciously. In doing that I believe I am helping people to live right up to the last moment.

The appropriate use of Holy Scriptures and prayer by sensitive and well-trained clergymen can also be of inestimable value in the total ministry of the ill.

ER: The three of you have a similar concept of the role of the clergy in supporting a cancer patient. You help by supporting, encouraging, listening, empathizing, and giving both faith and hope to a patient, his family and friends. You absorb the anger of a patient. You can be trusted with confidences and yet remain unshocked and uncondemning.

Ritual is often followed in ministering to patients. Father Shanahan, do you still administer the last rites to a patient who is coming to the end of his life? If so, what effect does this have on him?

JS: There has been a change in the administration of the sacraments that makes them more meaningful. The Sacrament of Extreme Unction is now called the Sacrament of the Sick. It is administered frequently and quite normally when a person is ill but not about to die. Last rites is a term reserved for the use of the funeral liturgy.

ER: Rabbi Asher, how does the Jewish ritual help people to come to terms with grief?

JA: As with every aspect of life, Judaism's rituals seek to provide outlets for emotions rather than submerge them. Our tradition understands the immediate response to the crises we experience and seeks to vest them with meaning in the context of our relationship with the divine. Thus when death comes the family's anger, its total withdrawal, is acknowledged. Certain normal religious functions are suspended. In our anger, we can hardly be expected to praise God. After the funeral the family remains at home for seven days, desisting from its regular habits and allowing friends to come to the house for communal prayer rather than going to the synagogue. After that week, and until thirty days after the death, normal activities are resumed, while some personal habits are still restricted, for which one would have no inclination anyway. For the ten months following, one does not engage in any activities that might be interpreted as unduly entertaining or engaging in levity. Eleven months after death, family and friends gather to consecrate a memorial at gravesite. This ritual demonstrates the "closing of the grave," a symbol that grief must now be set aside and we must come to terms again with life.

The most modern understanding of the grief syndrome acknowledges stages of emergence from it. Jewish ritual is designed to guide us from the most abject sorrow to renewed composure, allowing for time to bring its healing to the bereaved.

ER: Chaplain Laursen, what extra help can a person find in dealing with death and grief?

EL: Workshops, seminars, and retreats for clergy and lay persons are effective in helping them express their feelings and thoughts about death and grief. People of all ages have participated in these groups. Most of them have felt threatened at first, but after permitting themselves to become involved in the dialogue and in the process of reflection, they have found that some of their fears were lessened. These are subjects that we all prefer to avoid, but by bringing them into the open and confronting them we may be able to deal with death, and life, in a more realistic and wholesome manner. Members of communities in which such experiences take place have developed rich resources for ministering to one another when confronted by death and grief. They can be open with one another to a far greater degree than exists in the usual "denial" of real feelings.

I am convinced that this entire process of opening up to each other makes it possible for persons suffering all kinds of diseases of body, mind, and spirit to live more fully and to limit to some degree the destructive elements that threaten us.

ER: Unlike most of the people who support the patient and his family, the clergy continues to serve the family after the patient's death by helping them through the process of grieving. The ritual of a funeral service and a postfuneral meal for family and friends is as much a supportive gesture toward the bereaved as an opportunity to say farewell to the deceased. Following these brief distractions, the survivors may experience a deeper state of shock than they did at the time of death. The period of mourning begins. There is no way to shorten or lessen the grieving process, although it can be shared and the pain, in part, alleviated through the compassion of others.

Part VII
Grief and Recovery

19 · Grief and Recovery

Grief is a normal, necessary psychological process that helps a person adapt to the loss of someone he loves. The survivor is depressed and often withdraws from former interests, activities, and even friends. Grief is a very personal experience, and even among members of a family who lose the same person, the subjective experience of the loss will be different for each one. Losing a husband or wife is not the same as losing a father, mother, brother, or child. The closer the relationship, the greater the loss.

For an adult the psychological work of grief is connected with remembering and reliving the experiences he shared with the person he has lost. Grief is not a consciously determined task; rather, it is set in motion automatically and proceeds at the rate that is *bearable* for the individual. Grieving is painful because, as one remembers good times as well as bad, the very process of remembering requires a continuing recognition that the person he loves is not there now.

Grief involves intense mental anguish, remorse, and sorrow. The outward behavior of grief is identical to depression. But these are mere words, and can in no way suffice to describe the deep emotional inburst of pain and shock experienced by a person who mourns. He has lost love, goals, friendship, security, none of which is immediately replaceable.

The depth of grief is unpredictable, because it reflects so many factors —the availability of support from family, children, and friends; culture, religion, degree of preparation for the event, and many others. And there is no universal approach to the process of grieving, although in our society many people follow specified religious procedures. Each of the major religions observes a degree of ritual, quite similar in format, when dealing with death.

As a physician who deals with these problems frequently, I try to prepare a patient's family and friends as well as possible for an antic-

ipated death. I do this by providing medical information and holding
family conferences on the patient's progress. Yet no matter how thoroughly I have prepared them, the family will still experience shock and
momentary disbelief when the death occurs. In addition, questions will
be asked and decisions required of them. Will there be a postmortem?
What funeral arrangements must be made? This is where I can be helpful, because at such a time those close to the patient are not thinking or
remembering clearly. If the disease was chronic, funeral arrangements
have often been completed, or at least initiated, by the family.

When the funeral is over, the family, as well as the members of the
medical team that has been involved with the patient, need time for
their sorrow to abate. At this time I usually write the family a letter
expressing both sympathy and hope for the future. I also review the
patient's medical problem and the therapy he received, and give pertinent autopsy information. This alleviates any questions or mis-
understandings among family members about what actually occurred,
especially in the final days, when their comprehension may have been
clouded by concern for the patient.

In my letter I also discuss the supportive role played by the family
during the patient's illness. In almost every case the care and assistance
given by the family, in the hospital or at home, has contributed to better
medical care for the patient, and I acknowledge the help they gave the
doctors and nurses. Finally I mention the normality of grieving, in
addition to reminding them that there will be a time when life will be
less painful. I may say, "Life will be very difficult following your loss,
yet with time, the assistance and support of your children and family,
and your own perseverance and courage, you will build a new life
that will have both happiness and quality." I also invite them to visit
me at any time if they feel I can help them with their problems of
readjustment.

During the first few weeks, phone calls, visitors, and cards of sympathy distract the attention of the grief-stricken. Then suddenly the attention diminishes and one is left alone with the problem of the future.
Often there is a denial of mourning, an attempt to hold back tears and
suppress grief. Crying is felt by some people to be a sign of weakness.

Sometimes grief occurs simultaneously with unrelenting depression,
in which the survivor becomes obsessed with his loss. When this happens, the crisis has become chronic and debilitating for the survivor.
His persistent, unremitting loneliness, helplessness, guilt, shame, and
anger may lead to a regressed state, in which case professional help
may be required to alleviate his problems.

In more normal grief, friends and other family members may try
to prevent the bereaved from living in the past. They may try to create

diversions to lessen his emotional suffering. These efforts are helpful and important. However, grief must be allowed to run its course.

In March of 1975 I invited Janet Segal* to the monthly conference with the Patient Service volunteers at Mount Zion Hospital. The topic was grief and recovery. After opening the meeting with some remarks on the mechanisms of grief and adaptation to loss, I asked Janet to describe her own experiences since Mort's death, one year earlier.

JANET SEGAL: It's hard to know where to start. During this last year I have had wildly fluctuating moods and attitudes and have been better or less able to handle what my life is now compared to what it was before. Mort and I were married almost ten years and had a blessed and easy life. Neither of us, by personality, lived in the future, and so our life together didn't end with many regrets about things we hadn't done or were waiting to do. So I would keep thinking about all the good things that had happened, but each time I did this—and it is still true today—I would have to face the fact that Mort is gone and will not be back. Our children, Josh and Rebecca, are now four and six; and the fact that they won't have the influence of this most remarkable man is still, and will probably always be, hard for me to accept.

I feel guilty because I complain. What we had in a relatively short time was probably a whole lot better than many people experience all their lives. It seems ungrateful to complain, but I do. I had thought I would go through a maturing process in my grief, and reach a point where I would face the fact of Mort's death and accept it graciously. It is just in the course of the last week, while talking to a friend, that I realize I'm not ever going to accept it. Never, never, never!

The last year has not been a completely sad year for me. I don't feel that my life ended with Mort's death or that good things won't happen, because they have, and I expected they would. Of course, there were the circumstances at the end of his life. All that he was going through, his suffering, was finished, and that was a relief. But, you know, I may live to be a hundred and twenty years old and have some wild life beyond anything I could imagine in the future—I think that's perfectly possible—but I will never—no matter what happens in the future—I will never be able to accept graciously that Mort died when he did, and how he did.

In the course of the last year, I have been through different phases of grief. The phases seem to be repetitive and very short. At times I can be overcome and almost nonfunctional with grief, sad thoughts, resentment, and anger. I wonder what I would be like if I didn't have the children to spur me to action and decisions and all the other things.

* Janet Segal, the widow of Mort Segal (see Chapter 5), works three days a week as an executive at a university.

I might otherwise have apathy or become one of those people who sit in the corner and put the drapes over their head and everyone would have to work to get me to move. The children saved me from that. They've also had a year of grieving and also have a lot of pleasant memories of Mort. Josh has always been able, without any concerted effort, to talk about Mort or refer to him, because Mort was a big person in our lives and is just naturally a part of our conversations, or record, or reference.

Josh will say, "Was that a car like Mort's?" or "Remember when Daddy took us here?" or "That's Mort's book." For me this has been helpful.

ER: The effect of a parental loss on children is deep. A few months ago, when I said good-by to Josh after a visit, he replied accusingly, "Ernie, you're not going to come back, just like my daddy."

JS: One thing I wonder about is my decision that the children should not see Mort after he died. They saw him the morning he died, and he was able to recognize them and talk to them and joke a little. Then they went out of the room and an hour later Mort died.

I did not have them come back and see Mort, and that is out of my childhood. I went to wakes with open caskets and remember thinking, "That's not what Grandma looked like," and for me that image remained. I felt this particularly for Josh and Rebecca. I did not want that image of Mort to be their most vivid memory of him, and I was concerned that it would be. They had known him such a short time and wouldn't have a store of images to draw on.

They have had a lot of questions since then, and I don't know but what maybe they would have felt better if they had seen him. But I made the decision for them. I still think it was right, but there is one step they can't quite put together. The last time they saw Mort, he was alive; and the next time, after I told them he had died, there was the funeral and his body was in a casket.

They have asked me the same questions many times since then. "Was Daddy's whole body in the box? Was he wearing clothes?"

Josh became very angry immediately after Mort's death. He had always been a friendly type, but then he was positively furious. His anger manifested itself with physical displays—throwing things, and so forth.

Rebecca knew Mort better. She reacted in a more "adult" way. She would be overcome with sobbing and want to talk, but was unable to talk because she just could not get the words out. As the months went by she became more able to say the words that Mort was dead and that she would never be able to touch him again.

Josh would on occasion say things like, "I wish I were dead, because if I were dead then I could see Daddy. Then I would be with Mort." I still don't think the children have accepted it either.

I had a lot of preparation before Mort died, because we knew it was going to happen and both of us talked about things and did some reading. What I'm trying to say is, I was better able to handle it because of the preparation.

Grieving is a selfish experience, but I guess, a necessary one. Grief is more intense the closer you are to the person who has died. You may have various parts of that relationship filled by other people, so that instead of one person, or one source, there are many sources. In that case the sum of the parts still doesn't equal the whole. Nevertheless, I've had a lot of support and for that I am very grateful.

The people who have helped me most through the grieving period are those who knew Mort, his complexities and his interests, because they know what he was really like. The support that comes from someone who knew the person—the talk, the conversation, the reminiscing, or the arguing about, or whatever—is most helpful. In the grieving thing it is sort of hard for me to hold myself together. It has been hard some of the time. Right now I don't think I have a lot left to give to someone else who is grieving.

ER: We all grieve after personal tragedies and losses. We progress from shock to recovery and, with time, move toward a new life. Anger and disbelief subside. Throughout the period of mourning, the concern and support of friends help the bereaved until a time comes when grief lessens. Life goes on, and the bereaved person joins in.

To the survivor grief may seem endless and recovery impossible. Nevertheless, a process does begin whereby grief and recovery occur simultaneously, in alternating patterns and moods. Of course, nothing is ever quite the same. The attitudes of the survivor may be permanently altered by his long acquaintance with illness, suffering, and death, and quite likely he will emerge from the ordeal a stronger, more mature person.

The means and length of time required for recovery will vary. Those who are alone will have a more difficult time and may need additional and continuing support from clergy, social workers, or the medical team to help them through their period of grief.

Slowly a new pattern of life evolves. At first the bereaved may feel guilty when he experiences brief episodes of enjoyment. To feel happiness may seem inappropriate, even traitorous. Yet it is these interludes of enjoyment that gradually create new hope. When they accumulate, they will coalesce into a vision of the future, and the survivor will be able to acknowledge emotionally what he always knew intellectually, that his vitality and involvement with others will return.

Little by little the painful memories of suffering and illness become less poignant, and it is easier to revive and enjoy thoughts of earlier, happier times. While cherishing these memories the bereaved may also derive courage from them by identifying with the positive qualities of the person who is gone. At the same time he will recognize with diminishing guilt that he has continuing needs of his own. This is the turning point.

There is no prescribed time that elapses before a grieving person begins to mobilize his interests and energy for the present and the future. There is no line of demarcation between grief and recovery. Old memories are kept alive while new ones are being created.

Conclusion

QUACKS AND UNPROVED TREATMENTS

Living with cancer creates a state of uncertainty. Some people have less tolerance than others to this and other stresses of coping with disease. Their anxiety may reach a level of panic at which ignorance, false hope, and despair lead them to search for quack cures. This can happen to patients who are receiving adequate support and treatment as well as those who are not. It can happen to the educated as well as the uneducated. A person who has cancer wants a cure, and when a cure cannot be guaranteed by standard medical therapy, he may go to any length to obtain a treatment that has not been sanctioned by any reputable doctor, researcher, or government agency. Sometimes he is encouraged by well-wishers who have no knowledge of the treatment of cancer. In any event, the patient convinces himself that such a move is realistic: it might work. In so doing, he often bypasses medically approved available therapies.

Hardly a week goes by without my receiving an inquiry about a new treatment for which spectacular claims have been made. These claims are usually in a newspaper or magazine article and are sometimes misrepresented by the editors to increase the sales of their publications. When this happens, the claims are often rejected by the researcher himself before they are brought to the attention of the scientific community.

Cancer quacks with their false cancer cures offer unproved methods of treatment that cost American patients between two and three billion dollars a year.* Some of these quack practitioners may sincerely believe their methods are effective; others are just capitalizing on other people's misfortune. Among the patients who refuse proved treatment and are

---

* Charlotte Isler, RN, "The Fatal Choice: Cancer Quackery," *RN Magazine*, September 1974, p. 56.

particularly vulnerable to the lure of the faith healer or the quack are those who have a difficult time accepting their diagnoses and the need for therapy. They often seek miracle cures and postpone entering treatment just long enough to allow their cancer to progress from potentially curable to incurable. Others who refuse standard therapy are misled by reports of the rare spontaneous remission or cure. Occasionally patients with benign chronic diseases such as arthritis or ulcers, or even with cancer, are cured without medical therapy. Medical literature documents these cases. However, the chances of such a cure are about as good as the chances of a cure from a faith healer or a psychic surgeon.

I have had several patients who visited local faith healers or flew to other cities and countries for illegal drugs. None of them has benefited from these desperate visits. Those who refuse or abandon standard therapy to pursue such delusive promises of cure are playing a dangerous game with their health. Many others who follow these promises are actually in good health and are, therefore, undergoing undue anguish. They have lumps or pains that have never been medically evaluated, yet are convinced they have cancer. They waste time, effort, and money seeking quack cures for a disease they may not even have.

Some of these treatments and drugs, such as Laetrile, are available in many parts of the United States, in spite of federal and some state laws banning their use. Laetrile is administered in a clinic in Tijuana, Mexico, as well as several other countries.* The Pure Food, Drug, and Cosmetic Act, passed by Congress in 1931 and strengthened by the 1962 Kefauver-Harris Amendments, stipulates that a producer of a new drug (or treatment method) must prove that it is not only safe but also effective, if it is to be licensed for public use. The Act provides for strict controls over investigational and experimental drugs and the sale of prescription drugs. Unless drugs are approved by the Food and Drug Administration, they cannot legally be distributed through interstate commerce. It is a federal crime, reinforced by our postal laws, to advertise or ship such products. Nine states have similar intrastate laws prohibiting distribution and sale of unlicensed drugs and methods, but until more states reinforce the federal legislation, unproved treatments will continue to be promoted and sold. In the states that have not passed their own laws, ways have been found to circumvent the federal ban against false claims in advertising.†

* Laetrile is a drug derived from apricot pits. I have never seen a tumor reduction in a patient with proved cancer who took Laetrile with no other intervening treatment.

† Additional information regarding Laetrile and other unproved cancer therapies (Koch, Mucorhicin, Hoxey, Lincoln Staphage, Krebiozin, Bolen test, etc.) that have been banned by the FDA can be obtained from the Department of

I do have an occasional patient who visits a faith healer or buys Laetrile in addition to taking standard therapy. Although I neither approve of nor condone the use of Laetrile or any other quack treatment, I do not reject these patients for medical therapy, and I do, if requested, provide them with the available literature about the useless treatment. To argue with such patients is harder than asking them to change their religion.

When patients resort to quack treatments, it may be the fault of a doctor who has given little consideration to their emotional needs and has taken away their hope for improvement. People don't want to die without exhausting every possible means of cure, and when disease progresses and therapy is not succeeding, the resulting depression and anger can damage even the best relationship between a doctor and a patient. At that point the patient may blame his doctor for the medical failure and seek quack cures. At other times the breakdown in rapport between a patient and his doctor may be the patient's fault. A patient's cancer is his problem, and he should do what he can to cooperate with the doctor. An attitude of "You're the physician; you find out what's wrong without any help from me" reflects a patient's anger and frustration and discourages his doctor. The patient who accepts his part of the bargain in trying to control his disease, who cooperates with his physician and has confidence in proved therapies, will help his doctor and himself.

LIFE AND DEATH WITH DIGNITY

Dignity is an attitude and experience that a patient creates for himself and that is enhanced by the attitude of his family, friends, and his medical team. All of us are concerned with dignity in life as well as in death. The concept of death with dignity has been discussed in many recent publications and forums, yet many physicians are still not alert enough to this issue.

There is a level of life with dignity that is acceptable to everyone, but the cancer patient may gradually see that level recede as he experiences diminishing control over his destiny. His life is suddenly influenced by his doctors and the mechanical procedures of diagnosis and treatment in the office and the hospital. He may feel depersonalized

Public Health, Fraud Section, Bureau of Food and Drug Administration, 5600 Fishers Lane, Rockville, Maryland 20014. Up-to-date information can also be obtained from the American Cancer Society, whose committee on Unproved Methods of Cancer Management—composed of doctors, lawyers, representatives of governmental and health agencies, and laymen—meets twice a year to review material prepared by its staff.

by the medical routine. He is reduced to an object, a captive of the medical system. But however frustrated and desperate he feels, he waits for a reprieve and tries to remain hopeful. Time seems endless. It often appears to be a lonely, isolated world. A cancer patient's life revolves around X rays, shots, examinations, re-evaluation tests. He may be hospitalized several times. As soon as one problem is solved, another arises. His loss of privacy and of control of his present and his future may become more of a concern than dying. He often asks himself and his doctor, "Is life worth living if it has to be like this?" He continues to try because he wants to live, like all of us, but he has fewer options than the rest of us, and he may feel that he is a burden to his family and to society.

In the terminal phase of his disease, a patient may suffer indignities. Many of these can be minimized, and his emotional and physical suffering eased, through a good doctor-patient relationship. One of my patients in a terminal condition was paralyzed and needed total medical support, yet he married two weeks before he died, carrying out the plan he and his fiancée had made before he became ill. During the last two weeks of his life his depression was diminished and he enjoyed each day with his wife, family, and friends.

Because of the common idea that a hospital is a place to die, not to get well, patients often resist admission. It might be their last trip. Once they are in the hospital, preterminal patients are sometimes isolated from other patients and visited less frequently by their families and the medical staff. In addition to loneliness, they sometimes experience a loss of dignity in an intensive care unit with its IVs and tubes. They naturally wonder, "What price will I now pay for my survival?" Patients have the moral and medical right to answer that question for themselves.

They may answer it by deciding to spend their remaining days at home, where they will have more peace and be in familiar surroundings. With the aid of nurses and social workers, a doctor can take care of almost any problem at home. I recently made a house call to visit a terminal patient whose one request had been to die at home. He said, "I know I'm dying and I'm not afraid. Thank you for letting me come home." His pain was well controlled by injections given by his wife. Nurses and social workers visited him daily, but his wife was his main source of care, with our help and direction.

Other patients may feel more secure in the hospital, close to trained personnel and special equipment. Or they may decide that being at home would add too much to the family's physical and emotional burdens and thus, perhaps, to their own.

Major concerns at this time vary from patient to patient. Some worry about becoming addicted to narcotics. Others worry about suffering and dying alone. For many others the question of an afterlife is paramount. The medical staff and I do all we can at this time to protect a patient's dignity and offer him peace of mind.

The question of how long to continue treatment is inevitably a part of these considerations. Medical ethics has not yet evolved a complete answer to this question, and in the meantime the decision remains the province of the clinical judgment of the doctor. But often the patient and his family clearly express the hope that when the end is approaching, suffering can be minimized even at the cost of shortening life; requests for euthanasia are becoming more frequent. Implementing such requests is neither ethical nor legal, but under the official guidelines of current medical practice, maximum comfort with a minimum of suffering can be promised. And although a request for euthanasia cannot be granted, it presents the doctor, the patient, and the family with another opportunity to discuss their feelings about how to proceed. I have noticed that after a patient has made such a request, he very often has another brief period of remission and the opportunity for renewed closeness with those he loves.

The family often suffers more during the process of dying than the patient himself, who may have accepted his own death while those around him are unable to let him go. Instead of acceding to the patient's wishes, families sometimes encourage the doctor and the medical team to make further efforts, while they, in anticipatory grief, persist in their own supportive efforts. One must have compassion for these faithful family members who are losing a part of their life, and at the same time recognize that the effort to prolong treatment is of little value to them or the patient. If the family can be convinced, the provision of comfort is the best approach.

Even though a doctor sees and cares for many patients who die, he is still affected by a patient's death. He may have taken care of a patient for several years and feel the loss not only of a patient but also of a friend. I am often asked how I can continue in oncology because of the emotional strain. When several patients die in a short period of time, it does become difficult. However, more and more frequently we are achieving long periods of remission and actual cures. It is these successes that sustain me and other oncologists.

LIVING WITH CANCER

The purpose of life is to live. The role of the physician is to help a cancer patient maintain as normal a life as possible.

There is a myth that you will die if you have cancer. This is not true.

Today one-third of all cancer patients are cured. The other two-thirds can be treated, and the majority of these, although not cured, are active, productive people. The outlook for cancer therapy is hopeful. With advances in the field—the discovery of new drugs, new combinations of drugs, and new techniques of administering them—better programs are being developed, especially in experimental adjuvant chemotherapy for cancer of the breast and colon and osteosarcoma. A cure for cancer is not just around the corner; the idea that a breakthrough is imminent is fallacious. It will take five or ten years before we can add other forms of cancer to those that are now curable.

The word "cancer" produces instant fear and visions of suffering or death; yet other diseases such as diabetes and those of the heart and kidneys may be far more serious and life-threatening than cancer if they are not treated. Even when they are treated, people who suffer from them are not cured. Their lives are in jeopardy unless their disease is controlled by treatment.

In the preceding pages I have described many different forms of cancer and their treatment. I have discussed the impact on a person of being told he has cancer, how he must grapple with shock, fear, and depression, and how these emotions can threaten him throughout the course of his disease. The patients whose stories are told here illustrate how they, like other people, differ physically and emotionally in the way their disease affects them, and why a doctor's approach to treatment must be flexible and adaptable to individual needs.

Having cancer often intensifies both problems and pleasures. People who seem to have a better medical response are those who have a good self-image, the support of family and friends, and the will to live. Many patients find it helpful to share their experiences with other patients, as well as with those close to them. It also helps a new patient to talk with someone who has experienced therapy and its side effects. For this reason I often ask a patient on chemotherapy to talk with another who is about to begin treatment. It may be good for both, and the decrease of fear and anxiety can increase a patient's potential for coping with his disease and his treatment.

Fear is present from the moment a person has reason to suspect he has cancer, and it may so paralyze him that he is unable to seek medical help. Nevertheless, early detection gives a far better chance for cure. This is one reason why, in the 1970s, we can cure one in three patients. Forty years ago we cured one in five.

Cancer is no longer a disease in which the surgeon plays the major role. In medical centers throughout the world cases are being evaluated and staged through a cooperative approach that includes the medical oncologist, the surgeon, and the radiotherapist. A comprehensive review by this team of doctors, and possibly outside consultants, results in a recommended treatment plan. The attitude of the medical team is essentially that, no matter what the stage of disease or gravity of the problem, treatment is possible; symptoms can be alleviated and side effects controlled.

A patient should be able to talk to his doctor on a one-to-one level. The doctor should take the time to explain the diagnosis, its meaning, and the chances for cure or control of the disease. He should explain the tests and treatments the patient will undergo, and how pain and discomfort can be controlled by medication. Finally, he should assure the patient of his ongoing medical and personal support. A cancer patient should have this personal care. He does not want to be part of a medical therapy production line where two hundred other patients, in all stages of cancer, are seen daily. Many patients rightfully have difficulty accepting a doctor or a system that depersonalizes care. They want time from their doctor, empathy, candor, and a feeling of mutual trust.

Most of all, a doctor can help keep hope alive for the patient and his family by helping them to mobilize their own resources. Hope is defined according to the reality of the disease. A patient who has achieved a remission will hope for a prolonged reprieve and, with time, a cure. A patient like Ellen Abbott, who knows she isn't going to win her battle against cancer, may still be able to say, as she did, "Each day, week, and month that we pass—particularly if I am free to enjoy life during that time—is a victory." Such will to live and endure prolongs life and hope. A patient in the final stages of disease also has hope—for peace of mind and freedom from pain.

Many books have been written about death and dying. I am concerned with the living patient and his search for a way of life, even if it is altered by his disease, in which he can accomplish his goals and achieve some happiness. This is feasible. Most people who have cancer are continuing to work, to take vacations, to enjoy their friends and families, and to do many of the things they most want to do in life.

Many patients tell me that living with the uncertainties of cancer makes life more meaningful, intensifies their appreciations, and eliminates much hypocrisy. When they can reduce their bitterness and anger toward their disease and accept the inevitable compromises involved in living with cancer, they discover they need not be devastated by it. For others, the uncertainties and emotional stresses predominate and discourage efforts to enjoy life.

All cancer patients must live with their disease. The decision on how to approach the problem is theirs. With the proper support from family, friends, and the medical team, and with their own inner resources of courage and hope, they can continue to live a meaningful life.

> Choose life—only that and always, and at whatever risk. To let life leak out, to let it wear away by the mere passage of time, to withhold giving it and spreading it, is to choose nothing.
>
> ANONYMOUS

Appendixes and
Glossary of Medical Terms

Appendix I · A Patient's Bill of Rights

The American Hospital Association presents a Patient's Bill of Rights with the expectation that observance of these rights will contribute to more effective patient care and greater satisfaction for the patient, his physician, and the hospital organization. Further, the Association presents these rights in the expectation that they will be supported by the hospital on behalf of its patients, as an integral part of the healing process. It is recognized that a personal relationship between the physician and the patient is essential for the provision of proper medical care. The traditional physician-patient relationship takes on a new dimension when care is rendered within an organizational structure. Legal precedent has established that the institution itself also has a responsibility to the patient. It is in recognition of these factors that these rights are affirmed.

1. The patient has the right to considerate and respectful care.

2. The patient has the right to obtain from his physician complete current information concerning his diagnosis, treatment, and prognosis in terms the patient can be reasonably expected to understand. When it is not medically advisable to give such information to the patient, the information should be made available to an appropriate person in his behalf. He has the right to know by name the physician responsible for coordinating his care.

3. The patient has the right to receive from his physician information necessary to give informed consent prior to the start of any procedure and/or treatment. Except in emergencies, such information for informed consent should include but not necessarily be limited to the specific procedure and/or treatment, the medically significant risks involved, and the probable duration of incapacitation. Where medically significant

* Approved by the House of Delegates of the American Hospital Association, February 6, 1973.

alternatives for care or treatment exist, or when the patient requests information concerning medical alternatives, the patient has the right to such information. The patient also has the right to know the name of the person responsible for the procedures and/or treatment.

4. The patient has the right to refuse treatment to the extent permitted by law, and to be informed of the medical consequences of his action.

5. The patient has the right to every consideration of his privacy concerning his own medical care program. Case discussion, consultation, examination, and treatment are confidential and should be conducted discreetly. Those not directly involved in his care must have the permission of the patient to be present.

6. The patient has the right to expect that all communications and records pertaining to his care should be treated as confidential.

7. The patient has the right to expect that within its capacity a hospital must make reasonable response to the request of a patient for services. The hospital must provide evaluation, service, and/or referral as indicated by the urgency of the case. When medically permissible a patient may be transferred to another facility only after he has received complete information and explanation concerning the needs for and alternatives to such a transfer. The institution to which the patient is to be transferred must first have accepted the patient for transfer.

8. The patient has the right to obtain information as to any relationship of his hospital to other health care and educational institutions insofar as his care is concerned. The patient has the right to obtain information as to the existence of any professional relationships among individuals, by name, who are treating him.

9. The patient has the right to be advised if the hospital proposes to engage in or perform human experimentation affecting his care or treatment. The patient has the right to refuse to participate in such research projects.

10. The patient has the right to expect reasonable continuity of care. He has the right to know in advance what appointment times and physicians are available and where. The patient has the right to expect that the hospital will provide a mechanism whereby he is informed by his physician or a delegate of the physician of the patient's continuing health care requirements following discharge.

11. The patient has the right to examine and receive an explanation of his bill regardless of source of payment.

12. The patient has the right to know what hospital rules and regulations apply to his conduct as a patient.

No catalogue of rights can guarantee for the patient the kind of treatment he has a right to expect. A hospital has many functions to perform, including the prevention and treatment of disease, the education of both health professionals and patients, and the conduct of clinical research. All these activities must be conducted with an overriding concern for the patient, and, above all, the recognition of his dignity as a human being. Success in achieving this recognition assures success in the defense of the rights of the patient.

Appendix II · Informed Consent Form

DATE: _____ NAME OF PATIENT: _____

I, the undersigned, consent for Dr._____
and/or associates or assistants of his choice to perform the following
procedure upon me:

and/or to do any other procedure that (his) (their) judgment may
dictate to be advisable for my well-being.

The nature of the procedure has been explained to me and no war-
ranty or guarantee has been made as to the results.

With these conditions, I willingly volunteer to aid in the research
study but reserve the right to discontinue at any time and without the
necessity of giving a reason.

Patient's signature_____

Witness_____

Appendix III · The Living Will

TO MY FAMILY, MY PHYSICIAN, MY CLERGYMAN, MY LAWYER—

If the time comes when I can no longer take part in decisions for my own future, let this statement stand as the testament of my wishes:

If there is no reasonable expectation of my recovery from physical or mental disability, I,_____, request that I be allowed to die and not be kept alive by artificial means or heroic measures. Death is as much a reality as birth, growth, maturity and old age—it is the one certainty. I do not fear death as much as I fear the indignity of deterioration, dependence and hopeless pain. I ask that medication be mercifully administered to me for terminal suffering even if it hastens the moment of death.

This request is made after careful consideration. Although this document is not legally binding, you who care for me will, I hope, feel morally bound to follow its mandate. I recognize that it places a heavy burden of responsibility upon you, and it is with the intention of sharing that responsibility and of mitigating any feelings of guilt that this statement is made.

Signed: _____

Date: _____

Witnessed by:

_____

_____

Glossary

acute infection an infection of viral or bacterial origin that develops and progresses rapidly, as opposed to a chronic infection, which may have a prolonged course.

adjuvant programs the administration of chemotherapy to patients from whom all known cancer has been surgically removed. This may destroy small amounts of undetected cancer.

alkylating agents a family of chemotherapeutic drugs that combine with DNA (genetic substance) to prevent normal cell division.

amphetamines drugs that stimulate a patient's nervous system.

analgesic a drug used for reducing pain.

androgens male sex hormones.

anemia the condition of having less than the normal amount of hemoglobin or red cells in the blood.

angiogram the process of visualizing an X-ray image of the blood vessel through the introduction of a substance that renders the blood vessels radiopaque (capable of blocking X rays).

anticoagulants drugs that reduce the blood's ability to clot.

antimetabolites a family of chemotherapeutic drugs that interfere with the processes of DNA production, and thus prevent normal cell division.

arterial system a branching pattern of vessels by which blood is distributed from the heart to all tissues of the body.

arthritic disease a broad category of diseases that result in pain or decreased flexibility of joints.

atrophied withered or reduced in bulk.

bacteria one-celled primitive plant organisms widely encountered in nature, capable of causing disease in humans.

barbiturates a specific class of drugs capable of inducing relaxation, narcosis, sleep or unconsciousness.

BCG (Bacillus Calmette-Guérin), a form of the tuberculosis bacterium, used primarily for TB vaccination, which can act as an excellent stimulant to the immune system.

benign not malignant.

biopsy the surgical removal of a small portion of tissue for diagnosis.

blood chemistry panels multiple chemical determinations prepared by an automated method from a single sample of blood.

blood clot a solid composed of blood components held together by interlacing strands of fibrin (the major protein of blood coagulation).

blood count a laboratory study to evaluate the amount of white cells, red cells, and platelets.

blood transfusion the introduction of whole blood (red cells and/or plasma) into the circulation to replace blood lost or to correct anemia.

bone marrow a soft substance found within bone cavities, ordinarily composed of fat and developing red cells, white cells, and platelets.

bone-marrow examination the process of removing bone marrow from the cavity by withdrawing it through a needle for pathological examination.

Burkitt's lymphoma a lymphoma originally described in Africa as readily cured by chemotherapy.

cancer the proliferation of malignant cells which have the capability for invasion of normal tissues.

carcinoid a potentially malignant tumor arising in the wall of the gastrointestinal tract or bronchial tree, capable of secreting substances causing diarrhea, flushing, or rapid heartbeat.

cardiac of or pertaining to the heart.

cardiac arrest a situation in which the heart ceases to function.

catheter a hollow tube (rubber, plastic, glass, or metal) for introduction into a body cavity (e.g., the bladder) to drain fluid.

cell-cycle specific chemotherapeutic drugs that kill only cells which are in the process of division.

cervix the lower portion of the uterus, which protrudes into the vagina and forms a portion of the birth canal during delivery.

charged particles portions of an atom that are attracted to either the positive or the negative pole of an electric field.

chemotherapy the treatment of disease by chemicals (drugs) introduced into the bloodstream by injection or taken by mouth as tablets.

choriocarcinoma a carcinoma composed of cells arising from the placenta or, rarely, in the testes.

chronic defining a disease process that develops over a long period of time and progresses slowly.

cobalt, cobalt treatment radiotherapy using gamma rays generated from the breakdown of radioactive cobalt-60.

codeine a narcotic analgesic drug prepared from the stems of the opium poppy, used for control of pain and treatment of cough and diarrhea.

colostomy formation of an artificial anus in the abdominal wall, so the colon can drain feces into a bag (see *ostomy*).

coma a condition of decreased mental function in which the individual is incapable of responding to any stimulus, including painful stimuli.

consultation the formal process of soliciting the opinion of a specialist.

coronary thrombosis blockage of the arteries serving the heart muscle, resulting in death of a portion of the heart.

cyanotic a blue appearance of the skin, lips, or fingernails as the result of low oxygen content of the circulating blood.

cyst a fluid-filled sac of tissue; a cyst may be malignant or benign.

Demerol a potent synthetic narcotic analgesic related to morphine.

diagnosis the process by which a disease is identified.

diagnostic procedures studies designed to yield information about the nature and extent of disease in a patient.

digestive tract the esophagus, stomach, and intestines and colon, including such other organs involved in digestion as the liver and the pancreas.

diuretics drugs that increase the elimination of water and salts (urine) from the body.

DNA abbreviation for deoxyribonucleic acid, the building block of the genes, responsible for the passing of hereditary characteristics from cell to cell.

dolophine a synthetic narcotic (methadone) analgesic related to morphine.

edema the accumulation of fluid within the tissues.

electrocardiogram a method of evaluating heart rhythm and muscle function by the measurement of the heart's electrical impulses.

electrons negatively charged particles making up the outer shell of atoms; electron beam is a form of radiotherapy used for treating the skin.

enzymes proteins that assist the occurrence of specific chemical reactions; the increase of certain enzymes in the blood may be a measure of certain diseases.

estrogens female sex hormones.

euthanasia (1) an easy or calm death (Greek: *eu* = well, *thanatos* = death) (2) the act of causing death painlessly, to end suffering. The second definition is the one generally used in medical contexts.

excision surgical removal of tissue.

exploratory surgery undertaken to investigate a situation that diagnostic tests have failed to clarify.

foci in cancer diagnosis, minute deposits of cancer cells which are undetectable by ordinary methods of examination.

four-drug chemotherapy program, multidrug chemotherapy the use of several chemotherapeutic agents at one time to improve the chance of response.

gene a portion of DNA capable of transmitting a single characteristic from parent to progeny.

hemangiopericytoma a rapidly growing, highly malignant cancer arising from the walls of blood vessels.

hematologist a physician (internist) specializing in the study of blood diseases.

hematoma a blood lump in the skin following a local hemorrhage.

history and physical examination the routine by which information is obtained from the patient and his physical characteristics are assessed.

Hodgkin's disease a form of lymphoma that arises in a single lymph node and may spread to local, then distant lymph nodes and finally to other tissues commonly including the spleen, liver, and bone marrow.

hormonal anticancer therapy a form of therapy which takes advantage of the fact that certain cancers will stabilize or shrink if a certain hormone is added or removed.

hormones naturally occurring substances that are released by the endocrine organs and circulate in the blood, stimulating or turning off the growth or activity of specific target cells or organs.

hydration defines the status of the patient with regard to body water; he may be dehydrated, well hydrated, or excessively hydrated (edematous).

ice blanket a blanket cooled with ice water or a refrigerant on which a patient lies to reduce his temperature.

immune identifies the state of adequate defense against a particular infection or possibly against a certain cancer.

immunology the study of the body's natural defense mechanism and of the diseases that result from deficient or inappropriate defense responses.

immunotherapy a method of cancer therapy that stimulates the body defenses (the immune system) to attack cancer cells or modify a specific disease status.

inflammation the triggering of local body defenses resulting in the outpouring of defensive cells (leukocytes) from the circulation into the tissues, frequently with associated pain and swelling.

"informed consent" a legal standard defining how much a patient must know about the potential benefits and risks of therapy before being able to agree to undergo it knowledgeably with legal responsibility for the result.

infuse to introduce any liquid foreign substance into a vein or artery.

intern a physician in the first year of training following graduation from medical school.

internist a specialist in internal medicine, dealing with the nonsurgical treatment of diseases.

intestinal tract esophagus, stomach, small bowel, and colon.

intramuscular literally, within the muscle; usually refers to the injection of a drug into the muscle, whence it is absorbed into the circulation.

intravenous (IV) the administration of a drug or of fluid directly into the vein.

intravenous pyelogram the intravenous administration of a radiopaque dye which is concentrated and excreted by the kidneys, making the kidneys and drainage system visible with X rays.

irrigation washing with a stream of water or other fluid.

isotopic scan a class of diagnostic procedures for assessing organs (liver, bone, brain) in which particular radioactive substances are introduced intravenously; the relative concentrations of these substances are detected by their radioactivity, yielding information about cancerous involvement of specific structures.

jaundice the accumulation of bilirubin, a breakdown product of hemoglobin, resulting in yellowish discoloration of the skin and of the white portion of the eyes; this is indicative of liver disease or blockage of the major bile **ducts.**

Laetrile a cancer "cure" promoted by unethical practitioners and having no proved demonstrable value; otherwise known as amygdalin or vitamin B17.

laparotomy any surgical procedure that involves entering the abdominal cavity.

laryngectomy the surgical removal of the larynx, or voice box.

leukemia a malignant proliferation of white blood-forming cells in the bone marrow; cancer of the blood cells.

lobe a natural division or segment of an organ.

localized with reference to cancer, this means confined to the site of origin without evidence of spread or metastasis.

lucid alert and aware of one's surroundings.

LVNs licensed vocational nurses; technical functions which they may legally perform are limited.

lymph nodes organized clusters of lymphocytes through which the tissue fluids drain upon returning to the blood circulation; they act as the first line of defense, filtering out and destroying infective organisms or cancer cells and initiating the generalized immune response.

lymphangiogram a diagnostic method by which radiopaque dye is introduced into the lymph channels which drain tissue fluids to the blood circulation; this dye is filtered by the lymph nodes, making them visible on X ray, and cancerous involvement of lymph nodes is evaluated by this test.

lymphocytes a family of white blood cells responsible for the production of antibodies and for the direct destruction of invading organisms or cancer cells.

lymphoma a malignant, or cancerous, proliferation or lymphocytes or other cells in lymph nodes.

malignant having the potentiality of being lethal if not successfully treated. All cancers are malignant by definition.

mastectomy the surgical removal of the breast.

melanoma a cancer of the pigment cells of the skin, usually arising in a pre-existing pigmented area (mole).

metastasized, metastatic the establishment of a second site or multiple sites of cancer remote from the primary or original site.

modality a general class or method of treatment. The basic modalities of cancer therapy include surgery, radiation, medical (chemotherapy or hormonal) therapy, and experimental immunotherapy.

multimodality therapy the use of more than one modality for cure or palliation of cancer.

myelogram the introduction of radiopaque dye into the sac surrounding the spinal cord, a process which makes it possible to see tumor involvement of the spinal cord or nerve roots on X ray.

narcotics a legal term defining euphoric and analgesic substances whose use is closely regulated by the federal government; natural and synthetic relatives or morphine make up the major class of narcotics.

neurologic pertaining to the nervous system.

nodes see *lymph nodes.*

noncell-cycle specific chemotherapeutic drugs capable of destroying cells that are not in active division.

oncologist an internist who has subspecialized in cancer therapy and has expertise in both chemotherapy and the handling of problems arising during the course of the disease.

oophorectomy the surgical removal of an ovary.

opacity, opaque the property of being impervious to light or to X rays (radiopaque); the opposite of radiolucent.

osteosarcoma tumor of the bone.

ostomy a surgically created passage connecting an internal organ with the skin for purposes of excretion (see *colostomy*).

ovary the female gonad, responsible for the production of ova (eggs) and of female sex hormones.

Pap smear Papanicoulau smear, a screening diagnostic procedure for the rapid detection of precancerous and cancerous conditions of the cervix.

paramedical refers to skilled nonphysician personnel who participate in providing care.

Parkinson's disease a degenerative disease of the brain resulting in tremor and rigidity of the muscles.

pathologist a physician skilled in the examination of tissues and in the performance and interpretation of laboratory studies.

percodan a narcotic analgesic compound related to morphine.

perivascular about or surrounding blood vessels.

prognosis an estimate of the outcome of a disease process based on the status of the patient and accumulated information about the disease and its treatment.

progression the advancement or worsening of a cancer with respect to size.

promyelocytic a stage of acute leukemia.

prophylactic treatment designed to prevent a disease or a complication that has not yet become evident.

prostate an organ located at the bladder neck in males. It produces some components of the semen.

prosthetic an artificial structure designed to replace or approximate a normal one.

protons positively charged particles, which with neutrons make up the atomic nucleus.

psychosomatic pertaining to the mind and body, an affliction with emotional disturbance reflected in physical or mental components.

pulmonary embolus a life-threatening condition in which a blood clot becomes dislodged from a vein and travels to a branch of an artery carrying blood to the lungs (pulmonary artery).

radiation, radiation therapy the use of radiation for control or cure of cancer.

radical an extensive operation to remove the site of cancer and adjacent structures and lymph nodes.

radiolucent transmitting X rays easily (e.g., the lungs are normally radiolucent).

radiosensitive describes a cancer that responds readily to small dosages of radiation; the opposite is radioresistant.

regression the diminution of cancerous involvement, usually as the result of therapy; it is manifested by decreased size of the tumor (tumors) or its clinical evidence in fewer locations.

relapse the reappearance of cancer following a period of remission or absence of evident active disease.

remission the temporary disappearance of evident active cancer, occurring either spontaneously or as the result of therapy.

resection the surgical removal of tissue.

resident a physician who is undergoing specialized hospital training after internship.

residual disease, residual tumor cancer left behind following the palliative removal of cancerous tissue.

resuscitation, resuscitative a procedure designed to restore and sustain normal function in an individual who has undergone failure of respiration or of heartbeat.

reverse isolation isolation to prevent visitors or hospital staff from carrying an infection into a patient's room; gowns, gloves, and masks are worn by those who enter.

sarcoma a cancer of connective tissue, bone, cartilage, fat, muscle, nerve sheath, blood vessels, or lymphoid system.

scans see *isotopic scan.*

sciatic nerve a large nerve originating within the buttock and coursing down the back of the thigh.

sedatives drugs used to induce drowsiness or sleep.

seizure an abnormal discharge by brain cells resulting in involuntary movement, unusual behavior, or periods of unconsciousness.

semicomatose in a partial coma or state of unconsciousness.

sepsis bacterial growth within the bloodstream.

spleen an organ adjacent to the stomach, composed mainly of lymphocytes.

staging an organized process of ascertaining the extent of spread of a cancer.

STP a nonapproved drug that stimulates the nervous system.

subcutaneous cyst a cyst located beneath the skin, usually benign (see *cyst*).

suppository a drug administered by insertion into the anus, where it is gradually absorbed into the bloodstream; vaginal suppositories are used to treat local conditions and are not absorbed.

symptom a manifestation or complaint of disease as described by the patient, as opposed to one found by the doctor's examination; the latter is referred to as a "sign."

systemic disease disease which involves virtually all parts of the body.

terminal a condition of decline toward death, from which not even a brief reversal can be anticipated.

testicular mass a firm swelling involving a testis, or testicle, the male gonad.

therapeutic procedure a procedure intended to offer palliation or cure of a condition or a disease.

thoracic of or pertaining to the thorax, the chest—the rib cage and all organs within it.

toxicity the property of producing unpleasant or dangerous side effects.

tumor a mass or swelling. In itself the word "tumor" carries no connotation of either benignity or malignancy.

ulcer an erosion of normal tissue resulting from corrosive chemicals (i.e., acids), infection, impaired circulation, or cancerous involvement.

vasectomy the surgical interruption of the spermatic cords, the tubes that carry sperm cells from the testicles to the penis; the operation results in sterilization.

vital structure an organ whose unimpaired functioning is essential for life.

xeromammogram X-ray examination of the breasts by a new method that improves the detail representation of soft tissues and facilitates the diagnosis of minute areas of cancer.

About the Author

Dr. Rosenbaum, a hematologist and oncologist, is in private practice in San Francisco. At the Mount Zion Hospital and Medical Center, he is Associate Chief of Medicine and Codirector of the Immunology Research Laboratory. He is also associated with the Claire Zellerbach Saroni Tumor Institute of the Mount Zion Hospital and Medical Center, and the University of California Medical School.